SHAPE UP AMERICA!

SHAPE UP AMERICA!
A Diet for the New Era

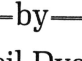by

Ceil Dyer

G.P. PUTNAM'S SONS
NEW YORK

Copyright © 1978 by Ceil Dyer

SBN: 399-12056-4

Library of Congress Cataloging in Publication Data

Dyer, Ceil.
Shape Up America!

1. Reducing diets—Recipes.   I. Title.
RM222.2.D94   1978   613.2'5   77-13627

PRINTED IN THE UNITED STATES OF AMERICA

Contents

6

Foreword

For millions of Americans, obesity is a painful fact of life. While most of the damage done by obesity is to one's ego and self-concept, there are diseases, such as maturity-onset diabetes, which appear to correlate directly with excess body weight. The emotional and physical pain of carrying excess weight forces many Americans to seek easy causes and easy remedies, which are not readily forthcoming. Therefore, the obese patients beseige doctors, looking for "glandular" causes, for occult kidney, heart, or liver disease that cause fluid retention and weight gain, or for metabolic defects that preferentially turn calories to excess fat instead of energy. For the vast majority of these patients who seek help there is no such easy answer. Most obese Americans are that way simply because they eat more food than they burn in energy expenditure.

Similarly, the multiple treatments available for obesity, both by the medical profession and lay organizations, attest to the fact that there are no simple, easy remedies. Appetite-control pills, thyroid hormone supplements, physician exhortations, rice diets, "fat farms," "fluid pills" and hormone shots have all been utilized in efforts to get patients to lose weight. Much more radical are the publicized intestinal bypass operations, the wiring together of jawbones and other "surgical tricks" to induce weight loss. The proliferation of diet books, diet clubs, behavioral-modification groups and recurrently published "best-seller" diet books all attest to the fact, painful though it may be, that there is no simple answer to the problem of obesity. For any treatment plan—be it medically sponsored or self-devised—to be successful and result in permanent weight loss, it is clear that modification of eating and daily-living habits must be instituted and maintained. Few of the fad diets and medically available remedies ever achieve this successfully. There has to be re-education to a new eating life-style in order for any person to successfully reduce his body weight and maintain for a long period of time this successful reduction.

In this book, Mrs. Dyer has provided a framework whereby, with diligent work and practice, the person with a problem of being overweight can re-educate his thinking about food and eating patterns and, with the help of recipes herein provided, retrain himself in cooking and eating habits so that the painful hunger of crash and fad diets can be avoided. The dietary theories and recipes given here represent a medically safe-and-sound approach that can help in gradually causing relatively painless weight loss with some assurance of maintaining that weight loss on a permanent basis.

DONALD K. WALLACE, MD

SHAPE UP AMERICA!

Introduction

It's long past time for a new deal in diet books. It's far too late for yet another easy-sounding but impossible (or even dangerous) series of half truths that leave you perhaps only a few dollars poorer for the price of the book but robbed, literally robbed, of your God-given right to a normal, healthy body by the almost-cruel process of yet another spate of empty words that promise the miracle they cannot and never will deliver. Oh, sure, the diet may work. In fact most of them do indeed work, and both author and publisher bask happily in the sunshine of yet another successful book. But for the millions who have happily (at first) shed the excess pounds the disappointment of their inevitable reappearance is a very real factor in what is rapidly becoming a national health problem. Consider the hopeful overweights who have trimmed off the 10, 15 or even 50 or 60 pounds; and note the very real pleasure and gratification they cannot help but feel; then consider the sense of defeat, the loss of the will to try again, when, within a brief time, these unwanted pounds are back. And back they will be, for until now practically no one has told the truth, the whole truth and nothing but the truth not about diet, but about *food*, what it can and cannot do to change not simply your body's shape, but your total well-being.

This is not merely another book of calorie-cutting regimens that will ultimately end in failure as they all do, but is truly a new deal, a new hand—an unvarnished, available, workable, lastingly effective way to regain your right (yes, *right*) to sane, healthful, delicious food. It will enable you to cease being the pawn of the food processor and the huckster, of the conscienceless commercialism that has taken over the very essence of life—the food we eat.

Further, this is a book for today, for now, not for a generation ago or a century ago when people lived totally different lives; when decent, nourishing food—delicious, healthful food—was not the rarity it has become, but an accepted, normal, day-to-day reality. A time when one simply purchased food with the confidence that the money spent at the grocery counter was spent to sustain and maintain a healthy, normal body.

Today overweight and all its depressing side effects, to say nothing of its downright danger to life itself, has become a national problem. It takes effort, knowledge and determination to maintain a healthy, slim body. But this book will give you the easy how, when and why to literally eat yourself thin and, not incidentally, enjoy the bonus of beauty that is the inevitable result of truly good food.

Does this sound like yet another so-called health-food book? It is not. The methods, ideas, menus and plans throughout the entire book are a practical "how to," the food largely available at conventional markets across the country, in every town and city of the United States.

This is a book on how to *cut* the cost of the food budget, not how to increase it; with, even more important, the ways and means to break the habit of spending useless dollars on non-foods, not simply by saying "Don't buy sugar-loaded soft drinks," but by showing how to have acceptable, cheaper and more delicious, substitutes.

The same type of "how to" is applied to snack foods, calorie-laden pies, pastries, so-called Danish, et cetera.

Equally important this book tells how to break the nutritionally impoverished yet ridiculously expensive "convenience-food" habit, and how to spend less time, not more, in the kitchen with far more delectable results.

1
The Motivation Factor

Many people, when discussing their overweight problem, have told me that, though they really wanted to lose weight, they were unable to "stay with" a diet—they simply did not have the willpower.

Dr. Donald K. Wallace, a specialist in nutrition and weight-loss problems at More Memorial Hospital in Pinehurst, North Carolina, believes that their inability is caused by lack of sufficient motivation. "It's not enough," he says, "to be just vaguely unhappy about those excess pounds. To lose them you first need a strong, compelling reason."

If your problem is the missing motivation factor, start here:

SEE YOURSELF

Who was it who said, "If we could but see ourselves as others see us"? No matter. But it is the sad and lonely truth that we rarely, if ever, see ourselves as we appear to others. Try it yourself. Walk to the nearest mirror. Unconsciously you pull yourself up and assume a pleasant expression. It's irresistible. All of us want to look well and we fool ourselves by this artificial, if comforting, means.

I can, however, tell you this—you fool only yourself. The rest of the world—your family, business associates, customers, friends, lovers and foes—see you as you really are and that "really" can often be the difference between success or failure in all aspects of your life. We are first, and sometimes always, judged by our appearance.

So try this: Turn away from the mirror. Relax. Now, quick, turn back and look fast. That is how you really look, for better or worse, until death or action on your part changes the inescapable fact of your true appearance. This is not to say that your unvarnished look into the mirror reflected a ghastly sight that made you turn away in shock, but if you—like me, only a few short years ago—saw a basically good body disfigured by fat—plain ugly fat—and you didn't like the sight, then start your motivation factor going now. Take a plain, hard, clear look in a full-length mirror each morning, right after you shower or bathe, *before* you get a stitch of clothes on to disguise (you think) what is really there.

I think it can trigger your desire to begin a new and lifetime pattern of eating that can slowly, but surely, rid you of excess weight and reshape your body more to your liking.

THINK YOURSELF THIN

Have you quit smoking? Do you know that the Surgeon General has determined that cigarette smoking is dangerous to your health? I'm sure you do—even if you continue to smoke. Well, everyone to his or her own poison, but I wish that statement would also appear in big, bold, red letters on every candy bar, so-called soft drink and package of junk food on our supermarket shelves.

They are, indeed, dangerous to your health and will keep you fat, fat, fat, yet hungry, dissatisfied and unhappy as long as you continue to eat such non-food.

If you are a junk-food or soft-drink "aholic" and your motivation to lose weight is weakened by these "sweet temptations," here's how to break the habit: Think before you eat; the sweet and junky food life may be killing you. The next time you reach for a candy bar, package of pretzels, or whatever, keep in mind that, even if they were manufactured under ideal conditions, they are loaded with questionable preservatives. How could they reach you were they not? They undoubtedly were shipped by truck over miles of superhighway and through air-polluted traffic fumes. Unloaded, they are placed, possibly for weeks before their purchase, on an open counter where dust and dirt filter through the attractive(?) wrapping. They are stale before you pick them up, but their staleness is masked by their sweetness or by a heavy hand of artificial flavoring. Do you really want to put that gooey chocolate-peanut concoction in your mouth? Think as you chew what each bite is doing to your irreplaceable teeth, how it is destroying the enamel, causing cavities. Do you really want to put all that non-food in your stomach? Your fine car gets only the best gas and oil. Isn't your body worth the same care?

KEEP THE RECORD STRAIGHT

If you are going to change your eating habits, starting tomorrow (but tomorrow is never today), keep a diary of every bit of food that you eat for a week. Don't cheat and forget that one chocolate mint. Buy a small book containing the calorie values of all basic foods. These books can be found at almost any bookstore and usually cost less than a dollar. Note the calorie total of each item, each dish—an approximate count will do for our purpose.

Now, go back and place a red check beside all of the high-calorie, low-nutrition foods that you ate, and ask yourself: Were they really all that good? Add up the number of calories you could have easily done without, those you wouldn't really have missed. It's a safe bet to say that it is those totally unnecessary calories that are keeping you fat. If they were subtracted from the week's intake, you wouldn't lose anything but unwanted pounds plus that pasty puffy complexion that is also the inevitable result of a diet rich in non-foods.

PROCEED AT YOUR OWN RISK

If your motivation for losing weight is not sufficiently strong to stir you into action, make a list of all the things you want—a better job, more money, someone to share your life with, a more youthful appearance, better health, more fun in your life, or whatever—then go over that list carefully and ask yourself: "Is overweight, bad skin, bad teeth, or lack of vitality slowing me down or actually making my goals unobtainable?" I'd say that ten times out of ten it is. The best jobs are more likely to be given to the most attractive, though otherwise equally qualified, people. Fat and unattractive people are less likely to find a desirable marriage partner. And as for falling in love with someone who is overweight—it's just slightly embarrassing, isn't it? Overweight detracts from your looks, makes you appear older, can—and usually does—undermine your health.

IF ALL ELSE FAILS

Attend the funeral of an overweight friend. Fat people die sooner than thin people. It's a proven medical fact.

OVERWEIGHT SAPS YOUR VITALITY

Vitality is literally the spice of life and vitality is directly related to what you eat.

Louise Dahl Wolfe, the famous photographer of World War Two fame, now retired and in her late sixties, has the figure and face of someone twenty years younger. No, not just the figure of one twenty years younger; she really has the body of someone in her twenties. Why? Simply because she has for years kept to a pattern of life that has proved to be a virtual fountain of youth. She, indeed, has the vitality of youth and it is a direct result of what and how she eats and drinks. No hard liquor at all, but wine with lunch and dinner.

Breakfast is fresh fruit and milk with a liberal sprinkling of wheat germ, a bran muffin or slice of wholewheat toast; coffee perhaps but more often tea. Lunch is a high-protein shrimp or egg salad, or perhaps a liver-pâté sandwich accompanied by a glass of wine. Dinner is usually simple broiled fish or chicken, or sometimes calves liver with a fresh vegetable, a glass of wine and then a lovely ripe piece of cheese with equally delicious ripe fruit for dessert.

I asked her how she established such a pattern and her reply was a revelation of what the right food can do for one.

"It was during the war years," she replied. "I saw so many people who had come out of concentration camps, how swollen and distorted their bodies were from lack of proper food, and I determined to keep the good body God gave me and respect the need I had for sound food. I simply will not insult myself by improper eating."

Maybe that is the key to motivation. You don't really want to insult yourself, yet bad eating habits and junk food *are* insults. Think about it. If you realize what you are putting into your body, you will not be prone to drink that soft drink, snack on cake, candy, et cetera, or have that cocktail for that matter.

One of the ways I found to teach myself to eat properly was to think of food and its origin. A piece of fresh fruit, grown in the open air and sunshine, is certainly more appealing than a slice of ersatz cake or a candy bar manufactured who knows where and under conditions that are more often than not unsanitary at best. If you really think, you won't be tempted to eat the wrong food.

Even a homely man or woman can be attractive. Overweight is a distortion, but one that can be easily and safely corrected. The bonus of a good skin, healthy hair and strong, handsome fingernails is free. Ask yourself simply this: Do I have pride in myself? For this single factor can provide the strongest motivation of all. Once you do realize that you want to take pride in yourself, you will have the enormous satisfaction of seeing the unwanted pounds slip away. You'll find it easy to keep to a sane, sound way of eating and you won't want to go back to bad-for-you food. To get started, envision how you want to look. Get a mental picture of yourself free of ugly overweight and keep it firmly in mind. It's simply a matter of determination and knowledge of what really good food is and how to enjoy it all the days of your life.

I have a friend who is not a pretty woman. In fact, when you analyze her face, it is really a bit ugly, but you are not aware of it in her presence. She gives the impression of being most attractive. Though into her fifties, she has a size-8, well-proportioned figure and she is always immaculately groomed. The combination gives an illusion of attractiveness.

I asked her how she had achieved this; the honesty of her reply surprised me: "I always knew I was homely. In college I really suffered from loneliness and I realized I would have to work harder than most girls to get what I wanted. I resolved then and there to have and keep a good figure and to maintain a super well-groomed look. It has worked for me. I have what I wanted. I love my job and my husband. I'm very lucky. I wish every unattractive woman would realize that one's looks are what one makes them."

Someone years ago coined the phrase "the Beautiful People," and there is a breed of Beautiful People whose lean bodies, glowing skin and luxuriant hair set them apart from the average. How do they do it? It sounds trite to say it's the food they eat, but this is the truth. What makes them so careful of what they eat? I think it is pride. They are proud of the way they look and they are determined to keep their good looks. Often the pressure of hard sell does tempt all of us to divert our appetites to useless calories. Consider the endless hours of television commercials devoted to hamburgers and soft drinks, but when you think about it—and I mean really think—how much more satisfying is a glass of fresh grapefruit juice than a sugary-sweet cola drink. The grapefruit juice can actually help you lose weight, while the soft drink can only add waterlogged pounds that take tremendous will power to get rid of. It's not worth it, is it?

Another factor that can trigger your determination to get rid of unwanted pounds is to go shopping for clothes. The most attractive dress or the best-looking suit can be a disaster on an overweight body. The man who finds it hard to tie the laces of a handsome pair of new shoes, the woman who discovers that a new skirt bags and sags because she does, will find a strong impulse to change bad eating habits for new ones. When you have a lean, trim body, just about anything looks great. Inexpensive blue jeans look marvelous on a slim figure; they are a disaster on a fat backside.

The main thing is that it's so easy to get in shape and

stay that way. The right food and a moderate amount of exercise will do the trick. You have to want to, of course, but I can give you another idea that will reinforce your desire for a lean, trim body. It's as simple as this: Look around you. That's right. Look at the overweight slobby people you see every day, their complexions pasty and dead-looking, their hair lackluster, their bodies ungainly with surplus fat. You don't want to look that way and you need not. If you realize that you can have what you want, not by starvation diets, but by sound nutrition, eating deliciously but sensibly, it becomes a form of mild insanity not to do so.

2
Basic Principles of Dieting

Are you dieting yourself fat? No, it's not a crazy question. You, like thousands of other people, may be literally dieting to gain weight. How? By going the seesaw route of a crash diet for two weeks, then back to the same old eating habits, putting back on the 4 pounds you lost plus 1 or 2 more. Then grapefruit and lamb chops again and off with 4. Then back to "normal" and gain 5. Result: a total 2-pound gain and four weeks of misery.

Few people have the willpower to stay on a conventional low-calorie diet for more than a few weeks and, as soon as they return to a "normal" diet, back comes the lost weight. The sad thing is that it is all unnecessary. Any normal person can lose weight safely and sanely by the very simple process of eating fewer calories than the body can burn up. The trick is in knowing how to make such a diet so delicious and satisfying that there is no desire to overeat. But there are other dimensions that have been largely ignored yet that remain important factors in weight loss. Simply this:

YOU CAN CONTROL YOUR APPETITE BY WHAT
YOU EAT. YOU CAN EAT FOODS THAT WILL HELP
YOU LOSE WEIGHT—FOODS THAT FLUSH OUT
EXCESS WATER THUS ELIMINATE POUNDS

How do I know this? By hard-won personal experience. A broken hip and the subsequent six months of inactivity left me at a dismal 154 pounds, up 26 pounds from my normal 128. Now, I like to eat well. I love to cook and I make my living writing cookbooks. Therefore all of the crash diets, whatever their name, made me totally miserable, and one, the high-carbohydrate version, made me literally sick. Happily, having some knowledge of food, I began to experiment.

First with how to cut calories from really great food.

Second with how to *combine* foods that would trigger both loss of weight and loss of excess water.

To say that it can be done is an understatement. You can eat wonderfully good, delicious, satisfying, nutritious meals and lose weight. Now, at a happy 126 pounds, I have proven it to myself and any normal, healthy person can do the same.

The food facts, the recipes and, equally important, the menus that follow will show you how to take off your unwanted pounds. They will prove to you what I have learned: It's not what you don't but what you *do* eat that determines weight loss or gain.

You can eat almost any food that you like and still lose weight. Rich-tasting stews, pasta dishes, potatoes, and even sweets can appear regularly on your menu *if* you understand how to cut calories from such foods without eliminating flavor and appetite satisfaction, and *if* you know how to combine them in menus that make it relatively easy to lose. That is what I have done here.

No one ever suffered from a dinner of sautéed chicken with mushrooms, parslied rice and fresh asparagus, ending with Bananas Flambé (see p. 225). Or what about avocado stuffed with shrimp salad for lunch? Perhaps the choice for tomorrow's dinner is Beef Bourguignonne followed by ripe pears and cheese. Sounds good, doesn't it? Yet all three menus contribute to effective weight loss. The trick is to eliminate all animal fat from both the chicken and beef dishes and use the pure protein of bones plus puréed fruits or vegetables to thicken the sauce. The plus factor of greatly enhanced flavor is free.

Or perhaps what you would really like is a creamy big baked potato. Have it with a broiled lamb chop or, even better, with a slice of sautéed calves liver liberally sprinkled with parsley and accompanied by a broiled fresh peach half. Dessert can be a delicate coffee-chocolate mousse.

Sounds ridiculous? Not at all when you understand the chemistry balance and the satisfaction quotient from any of these random menus.

High-protein count lessens your desire for too much high-carbohydrate food as well as oversweet desserts. The beef and chicken recipes step up the protein while eliminating fat. You can eat even a fairly generous portion and still lose. The Shrimp-stuffed Avocado, using Yogurt Mayonnaise (see p. 63) is a literal powerhouse of top-quality protein, vitamins and minerals, while weighing in at only 240 calories. Furthermore, avocados are high in appetite satisfaction and contain pure unsaturated oils to help the body burn fat.

As for the potato—stuffed not with cream and butter but with cottage and Parmesan cheeses—it is a sinfully rich-tasting but low-calorie transformation of this much-maligned vegetable that is, in fact, a rich source of vitamins and minerals, including the invaluable potassium that helps the body to eliminate excess fluid.

Note carefully the BALANCE of each menu. The low-fat high-protein chicken is served with low-calorie parslied rice and asparagus. Both parsley and asparagus are highly effective diuretics, flushing the body of excess water and toxic wastes. The bananas, prepared with lemon juice and honey, contribute vitamin C and a liberal supply of potassium.

Parsley is again used with a lavish hand for our Beef Bourguignonne and the potassium content and fruit sugar of the pears combined with high-protein cheese make for a true weight-losing combination. Again we use parsley and add a broiled peach half to our third menu for the same two-way effect. Finally the coffee-chocolate mousse is made not with cream but with yogurt; to my way of thinking it tastes even more delicious than the calorie laden variety.

But, you may scream, the trouble with good diet food is that it's fabulously expensive. Who can afford calves liver, lamb chops or chicken every night of the week? As for Shrimp-stuffed Avocados, who has the wherewithal? No wonder the so-called Beautiful People are almost always rich, rich, rich. Well, let me hasten to add that, if you eliminate soft drinks, candy, cakes, pies, doughnuts, potato chips and other ersatz snack foods from your grocery list, you may well find you are spending less grocery money even if you do treat yourself to the above-mentioned "luxury" foods. But no matter. The issue at hand is cold, hard cash and there is often simply not enough of it to cover the tab for liver, shrimp, lamb chops et cetera. Well, would you enjoy a sinfully rich-tasting supper of creamed chipped beef—smooth and delicious with the added taste appeal of chopped water chestnuts, the whole lavishly sprinkled with parsley and served on crisp toast? Or lowly tuna fish prepared the same way? The secret to both is the use of clear fat-free chicken stock instead of milk, extra butter and cream for superb flavor and even more superb high-quality, fat-burning protein.

For dessert? What about inexpensive canned figs, soaked in a bit of cognac or just plain brandy, then sprinkled with a trace of chopped almonds? That something as delicious as this can also be a highly effective means of ridding your body of waste and bloat may seem unlikely, but it is undeniably true.

Perhaps you would be in the mood for dinner Italian style. Select a generous dish of Eggplant Parmigiana enriched with two cheeses, chicken stock and a generous dash of Italian herbs. A glass of Chianti to accompany it, of course, and a creamy Zabaglione for dessert. See? Here again we substitute high-protein stock, cheese and eggs for high-calorie carbohydrates or fats. Added to this, the vitamin, mineral and roughage properties of fresh fruit and vegetables along with their laxative and diuretic effects that flush the excess fluids from the body.

But you simply haven't time (or money) to prepare things like shrimp salad for lunch. Jell a bowl of amber-clear chicken or beef stock, break it up with a fork and serve it in bouillon cups. Sprinkle it with parsley and top with a small spoonful of tangy yogurt. Accompanied by crisp whole-wheat wafers, it makes for a super lunch. Since this is on the light side, splurge a bit on wheat-germ Apple Betty for dessert, served with a small cup of fragrant black coffee.

Lest we forget the invaluable and versatile egg, dismiss that boogeyman of high cholesterol that food quacks have tried to associate with eggs. It's been completely, medically, disproven. A lunch of well-seasoned gourmet stuffed eggs on a bed of real Boston or Bibb lettuce is both delicious and satisfying. Don't make the mistake of substituting lifeless iceberg lettuce, which you will un-doubtedly leave untouched on your plate. Use crisp, green "vitality" lettuce, garnish your plate with crisp slices of unpeeled cucumber, cherry tomatoes and perhaps a few ripe olives, and you have lunch for a king.

One of the tricks for adding flavor and interest to diet meals is to include a piece of baked or broiled fresh fruit with your entrée. Broiled or baked halves of peaches or nectarines, slices of fresh pineapple, apples, et cetera, all add delicious contrast to meat, fish or chicken and step up the vitamin, mineral and roughage content which is what we are after.

Actually the formula for eating to lose weight is 1-2-3-4 simple. Faithfully followed it actually pares off the pounds and that's a guaranteed fact. Here it is:

FOR EVERY MEAL

High-quality protein
Lean meat, fish, chicken, organ meats, eggs, cheese, milk, cottage cheese, yogurt and stock.

Zero-saturated fats
Moderate saturated fatty oils.

Vitamins—minerals—roughage
Fresh fruits and vegetables of all kinds, the greenest crispest greens, the plumpest yellow squash, the reddest tomatoes, the most fragrant melons, peaches, berries, pineapples, apples and grapes and, of course, the green velvet avocado.

Finally the humble potato, best in its jacket, a bargain in vitamins, nutrients and taste satisfaction.

The plus of whole grain
Wheat germ, wheat wafers, thin-sliced wheat bread.

And lastly

A firm hand on the sugar control. Turn to "off" unless otherwise directed.

Easy, of course, but, more important, delicious and powerfully good for you, not only to shed pounds but to gain enormously in vitality. The sure plus of sheer joy of life is free.

To sum up: Plan diet meals for low-calorie density, meaning meals that are low in calories, yet sufficiently high in bulk to satisfy your appetite. Cut way down on fat from animal sources. You won't miss it. In fact use fats of all kinds sparingly. What you do use should be polyunsaturated, such as vegetable oil. Eliminate all possible over-processed and over-refined foods. Substitute instead fresh fruits and vegetables, lean meats, poultry, seafood and fish. Make every calorie add up to sound nutrition. Cut out, as much as possible, empty calories found in soft drinks and so-called snack foods, potato chips, crackers, candy bars, et cetera, in fact anything made with devitalized flour or refined sugar. They have no use whatsoever and can only add up to more unwanted pounds. But don't just eliminate calories; increase sound nutrition that acts to regulate body processes and properly utilize the food you do eat. Even slight deficiencies in any one vitamin or mineral can result in fatigue, irritability and nervousness, three of the major causes of compulsive overeating.

There you have it, the easy delicious way to lose weight—the two-way combination that pares off pounds without tasteless starvation diets, without the seesaw of lose and gain. In fact, I truly believe that, when you learn to cook and plan your menus around this new concept in food, you will never revert to calorie-laden, high-cholesterol fare again.

So come with me into the kitchen for a new dimension in dining. You have everything to lose.

DO YOU KNOW YOUR VITAMINS AND MINERALS?

Vitamins are essential to balancing any diet and, as such, they can have a positive effect on the body, causing natural weight loss while building general health and vitality. Most fast "faddy" diets suggest supplementing their ill-balanced regimen with vitamin and mineral capsules and, while they may be desirable or even necessary to prevent complete physical deterioration from such lopsided nutrition, they cannot and will not help you lose weight. Natural vitamins and minerals from the right foods can and will help you shed pounds. If you eat by the magical "Rule of Four" outlined above, you will obtain all the *natural* vitamins and minerals your body needs. Moreover, your body will assimilate them the way nature intended and no chemical substitute (for to be blunt that's exactly what most vitamin formulas are) can possibly substitute for what is in truth "the real thing."

The need for vitamins and minerals is exactly why you must eat a well-rounded diet to lose weight, for without the essential nutrients your body simply fails to perform. It cannot burn up even small quantities of food. We have all heard the timeworn joke about the fat woman who claimed she "ate like a bird." The sad fact is she probably did, poor woman, but her waterlogged, sluggish system simply refused to function. Unless you have some serious glandular malfunction that can be treated only by a skilled endocrinologist, a diet built around the "Rule of Four" will rid you of excess weight while providing you with the energy and vitality that, in itself, will cause even further weight loss.

The facts are very simple, as simple as putting gasoline in your car. The right fuel makes the motor "go," and, just as kerosene won't start your automobile, try as you will, the wrong food won't start your body motor. Every wrong bite you eat lodges as solid, ugly fat. Inescapable but true.

Put the money you have been spending on vitamin pills into the best, freshest food you can buy, and an occasional luxury like fresh lobster or crabmeat, or perhaps a small jar of caviar. It's not only more fun but far better for you.

A WORD ABOUT "DEMON RUM"

There is no doubt you can drink hard liquor in very moderate quantities and still lose weight while on a proper diet, but it is harder, much harder. As for continuing the martini lunch and the prolonged cocktail hour plus an occasional nightcap, forget it. That way you simply cannot lose weight, no matter how little you eat. What is even more important you stand to really wreck your health completely. Large quantities of alcohol rob your body of essential vitamins, particularly the B vitamin complex. Couple this with an inadequate diet and you not only stay fat, fat, fat, but you are courting disaster.

Poor nutrition, with its subsequent poverty of B vitamins and calcium, has a devastating effect upon the general nervous system. That shaky all-gone feeling, the frequent aftermath of "one too many," is a flashing red light of danger that means your system is depleted of calcium and B vitamins. The usual remedy of a "hair of the dog" only adds insult to injury. Anyone who has ever "tied one on" knows the calming effect of even one glass of milk, the poor misused body's pathetic reaction to even the bare minimum of calcium and natural sugar.

But why indulge at all? Alcohol is, of course, only a crutch and again, unless the problem is severe enough to warrant skilled medical help, such drinking is only a habit that's easy enough to break.

There are numerous reasons why people long for the icy martini or Scotch on the rocks, but two are the most compelling.

First is the need to relax and calm down. The nervous host or hostess on the threshold of a big and important party downs a "quick one" to steady the butterflies in the stomach; the apprehensive applicant for the "big job" finds that a vodka martini not only "leaves him breathless" but at least a bit more confident. The frazzled housewife or the harassed commuter, home at last, reaches for the day's-end Scotch and ice as a matter of course.

There is no real harm in moderate drinking, but what the seeker of steady nerves and a relaxed attitude doesn't realize is that, while momentary relief may be the result, it is only a matter of time until the need for one drink becomes the need for two and then more. Actually these same people do not realize that their inability to cope with the natural irritants and minor crises of life is a warning that they are suffering from severe nutritional poverty.

If all this sounds depressing, be of good cheer, for the cure is readily and pleasantly at hand. When we are starved for esssential vitamins and minerals, the nervous system is the first to react. Lack of calcium, for example, can be so severe as to cause literal symptoms of delirium tremens with its miserable shaking and shivering. Less violent but equally depressing effects are nervousness, irritability and inability to concentrate. For many people the cure has become a couple of drinks. Unfortunately this is like putting a penny into a blown fuse; the current goes back on, but the house is likely to burn down.

Instead try making a conscientious effort to step up your intake of foods rich in vitamin-B complex and calcium. Now if this sounds like a dreary substitute for a pleasant cocktail hour, it isn't. Try a slice of really great pâté on crisp Melba toast accompanied by a glass of chilled white wine. Or whip up a zesty dip from yogurt combined with grated onion, Tabasco and Worcestershire sauces to accompany the hors d'oeuvre tray of crudities—crisp, raw vegetables that have been well iced in salt water. With them, an aperitif, such as dry vermouth on the rocks.

Switch from a Scotch-and-soda nightcap to milk well laced with Cognac, a drink that would put a nervous tomcat to sleep.

Moreover, you can step up your B-vitamin intake with what I call my super breakfast. It's simply any fresh fruit I can lay my hands on—berries, peaches, bananas, whatever—plus a generous tablespoon or so of wheat germ, topped with plain yogurt. If you simply don't like plain yogurt, mix up your own combination of fruit flavors. I like apricot yogurt with peaches or bananas, boysenberry with any fresh berries. It tastes great, especially with a steaming cup of black coffee and it's low-calorie delicious powerhouse.

It is an established fact that, as you increase your nutrition, your desire for alcohol automatically diminishes. This is not to say you either should or will give up alcohol completely. Fine if you do—you have nothing to lose but excess poundage—but it isn't mandatory. A civilized glass of wine with a good meal is one of the pleasures of life and a chilled aperitif can be an enjoyable social end to a busy day. You should, however, put alcohol, like sugar, in its place as a pleasant "sometime thing," not a necessity.

The second, perhaps less important, reason for drinking is, for a lot of people, plain, simple boredom. The endless routine of their day is broken by the cheery cocktail hour and there's no harm in that. But if the cocktail hour stretches to three or four drinks, and if the subsequent repetitious television entertainment requires a stiff drink to dull the sensibilities, then I say, "Find a better use for your time."

No matter what the excuse may be, let nothing stop you from finding some pre-dinner activity that will take your mind off the boring day. It can be in the form of a leisurely late-afternoon walk. There's no better time for an hour's ramble *alone,* whether it's on a country lane or a city street. Late afternoon is a peaceable time. You'll come back refreshed, ready for the *one* cocktail before dinner with no need for a repeat performance. Or, if you are a tennis buff, try a short game before reaching for the Scotch. Or go for a swim or even play a few holes of golf. There is simply no better way to shake off the cobwebs of boredom than by light but invigorating physical activity.

As for after-dinner imbibing, try getting involved instead. Turn off the insipid television in favor of a really interesting evening. Take up bridge, become an expert at needlepoint, volunteer for a hospital (they are desperate for after-sun-down help), join a language class, take rumba lessons—in short find something you like to do and *do it!* You'll not only enrich your life and banish boredom, but you will find interesting, new, vital people who will be involved too, and there's no better stimulus for anyone than joining an enthusiastic group who are doing what you are doing—making life fun again.

If all else fails, take the advice given earlier in this book: Look in the mirror. But do it first thing in the morning. Now, honestly, does anyone want the bleary eyes and puffy face that is the inevitable result of a "bit too much"? Not you; not really; not now; not ever.

3
How Much Food
Do You Really Need?

Calories are sneaky things. You can't see them until too many add up to too much—on you. They have a treacherous, mean little habit of piling up as the years go by. If you and 1800 calories a day were compatible at twenty, they will turn on you viciously and start putting pounds around your middle at age forty-five. It's not fair, but it's true that, unless you step up activity rather drastically, the rule, more often than not, must be: more years, fewer calories. Your only defense is to learn to cook less, better, to know your food and to practice constantly the high art of creative low-calorie menu planning.

You know better than I do how much you should weigh so that you look your best; neither a haggard, skin-and-bones diet-frantic fanatic nor a sluggish unhealthy old fattie—but trim and lean and healthy. The experts can explain the arithmetic that will get you there. It's simple and basic—and perhaps you know it, but it's sufficiently important to deserve a review.

HOW TO FIND YOUR CALORIE LEVEL TO LOSE WEIGHT OR TO MAINTAIN AN IDEAL WEIGHT

Decide on your ideal weight. Be realistic. Much depends on your bone structure and type of build.

BASIC CALORIE ARITHMETIC

A calorie is simply a measure of the energy a food will give.

Balancing your calories is no more difficult than balancing your checkbook. Think of your body as a bank. You may not have a reserve in the latter, but you do in the former. Everyone has a certain calorie reserve (they are stored in the body as fat). If deposits and withdrawals are equal, the reserve remains the same. When more calories are withdrawn than deposited, the reserve diminishes (you lose weight). Calories deposited and not withdrawn increase the reserve (you gain weight).

DESIRABLE CALORIE INTAKE

Multiply your ideal weight by 15 if you are moderately active, by 20 if you are very active. The result is the number of calories you will need each day to maintain your ideal weight.

If you need to lose weight, subtract 500 to 1,000 calories per day from the number of maintenance calories. The result will be the number of calories you can consume each day and yet lose weight. Don't let the number of calories go below 1,000. You need that many to obtain nutrients essential to your health. There can be no beautifying effect from a quicky starvation program that will leave you depleted and robbed of your health.

4
Easy Ground Rules for Calorie Cutting

(*Without* cutting down on food portions)

The following paragraphs will tell you how to eliminate concentrated, fattening calories that you don't want, don't need, in fact shouldn't have and will never miss.

ELIMINATING THE FATTENING PART

What's the most fattening food you can possibly eat? The answer may not be what you have been led to believe. It is not pies, cakes, cookies, or candy and such, but fat. That's right. Fat makes fat fastest. Animal fat is the subject. At a hefty 126 calories per tablespoon this fat adds up fast and usually (always is probably the more accurate word, but an author must protect herself) proves to be, tablespoon for tablespoon, the most fattening part of your meal.

True, some fat is needed in every diet for general health as well as for an aid to weight loss, but the fat needed is the kind that comes in the form of natural vegetable oils. The kind of oil you use (I hope) to make salad dressing, and a small portion (1 to 2 tablespoons) is all that is needed each day.

What you don't need and—what you can live longer, healthier and slimmer without—is the greasy, heavy, fatty, fattening, hard animal fat found not just around the edge of a steak but in the usual soups, stews and meat-based casserole dishes described in almost every American cookbook. The tag line to such recipes almost always is: "Skim off surface fat and serve." But, you see, the truth is that only a small portion of fat will rise to the surface of any hot liquid, and that, of course, is why such dishes are prohibited on the usual low-calorie diet—and here again is the reason such calorie-restricted diets don't work. It's hard to give up this type of food. It tastes so good. We miss such dishes and eventually we say "What the hell!" (or less profane words to the same effect). "I want something rich-tasting—a good rib-sticking stew—a 'dishy dish,' as my English friend calls it—and I can no longer do without! I can't continue to give up all such food. ..."

Of course you can't. But ...

There is a way around this stumbling block to a weight-loss problem.

Abstinence is not necessary. You can have your rich-tasting soups and stews, as well as your sauces and gravies if you eliminate the fattening part—in other words the fat—all of it—before the dish comes to the table.

Sounds complicated? It is not. I've been doing it for years and I assure you it is simple, easy and makes good common sense too. Fat doesn't really taste good. It adds nothing but calories to a dish. In fact it actually detracts from the flavor. Don't believe me? Well, try this: Eat one—just one, more is too horrible—teaspoon of cold congealed fat, and not only will you know I speak the truth, but you will also swear off all animal fat for the rest of your life. What's more you'll agree with me and a fast-growing number of slim-minded gourmets that a dish—non-fat—is not only improved but can be enjoyed fully because there's this bonus: the enjoyment is without fat-minded guilt.

THE SAME FORMULA FOR REMOVING ALL FAT FROM ANY MEAT-BASED SOUP OR STEW—OR ANY MEAT SAUCE OR GRAVY—CAN BE USED FOR ALL RECIPES OF THIS TYPE, INCLUDING THOSE OF YOUR OWN INVENTION. IT IS NO MORE COMPLICATED THAN THIS:

SOUPS AND STEWS

1. Brown the meat if the recipe calls for doing so. Then pour off all rendered fat, and, with paper toweling, blot the meat dry of additional surface fat.

2. Add liquid (as desired or as recipe specifies) and seasoning, vegetables, such as onions, or garlic, plus dry or fresh herbs and spices. Simmer on top of the stove or bake in the oven until the meat is almost tender. Cool. Then refrigerate until fat has risen to the surface and congealed. Remove and discard congealed fat. (This happens when the liquid becomes cold and takes several hours.) If desired, do this part of a recipe one day ahead. You can double the quantities too and freeze half. Then use the frozen half as the base for a totally different second dish, adding other vegetables and different seasonings.

3. Heat the meat and liquid. Add additional vegetables or other ingredients as specified in the recipe and continue to simmer until meat and vegetables are tender. Correct seasoning and serve.

And that's all there is to it.

QUICK-COOKING MEAT DISHES WITH SAUCES OR GRAVIES

1. Prepare meat and sauce.
2. Pour off sauce. Cover meat and keep at room temperature. Place the container of sauce in a pan of cold water until sauce (or gravy) is cool. Place in freezer compartment of refrigerator until sauce is chilled and fat has come to surface. Remove and discard fat.
3. Reheat sauce. Add meat and reheat briefly in hot sauce. Correct seasoning and serve.

Hamburger

Yes, I know—it's one of the least expensive meats. It's quick-cooking and easy to prepare and besides you like it—but—*contrary* to what many low-calorie diet books imply—it's *not* low calorie. Far from it. Hamburger meat as you find it on "special" at your supermarket, already ground and wrapped in neat packaging, is *not* low calorie. Unfortunate, but true.

Hamburger meat must by law contain no more than one-third fat—but what butcher adds less to his own blend?

The only way to obtain lean—really lean—ground beef is to avoid prepackaged ground meat. Buy instead a lean cut of beef round or chuck. Have it trimmed of all visible fat and ground to your order.

Here's another time when "less" is "more"—to your weight loss advantage.

Consider the facts:

Prepackaged beef labeled "Hamburger" contains 25 to 30 percent fat, which brings it up to a whopping 344 to 399 calories per ¼-lb. serving. Prepackaged, so-called lean ground chuck is not far behind, containing (it can by law) 17 to 21 percent fat and weighing in at 290 to 316 calories per ¼-lb. serving. Custom-ground lean chuck, trimmed of all fat, drops to only about 180 calories per serving as it contains only 7 to 8 percent fat. Trimmed of all fat, lean ground-to-order round steak can be as low as 5 percent fat with a further drop in calories to about 170 calories for the same size serving. As you can see, what you know about ground meat and how you buy it can make a substantial calorie difference in an otherwise identical meat.

To cook very lean ground beef. Shape 1 lb. of meat into four very thin patties.

Place a heavy 10- to 12-inch skillet over high heat. Using a long-handled kitchen fork, rub the bottom of the skillet with a small piece of beef suet until it is covered with a thin film of rendered fat. Add the beef patties and sear them quickly on both sides. Now pour into the skillet—still over high heat—¼ cup of rich homemade beef stock (see recipe page 127-29) or half stock, half dry red wine, seasoned with a dash of red-hot pepper sauce plus a splash of Worcestershire. (If you have no stock on hand, use half water and half wine or good-quality brandy.) Cook at full boil until almost all liquid has evaporated. Season meat with salt and pepper—and there you have it! Nicely seared on the outside, faintly pink within—the best hamburger patties—or more accurately Haché de Boeuf—you'll find this side of Paris.

Serve open-face style on the bottom half of a lightly toasted bun with a little of the "pan juices" poured over, and topped with a thin, slightly heated slice of mild Bermuda onion and one of tomato, it's elegant as well as filling low-calorie fare.

FURTHER THOUGHTS ON CALORIE CUTTING WITHOUT CUTTING DOWN ON PORTIONS

Think veal. It is utterly delicious meat and—make a note, please—veal is one of the lowest-calorie meats you can buy, yet just as filling as high-calorie beef. For example, a 4-oz. rib steak can cost up to 475 calories, not to mention the high cost in dollars, while a veal cutlet of the same weight contains no more than 190 to 200 calories. Broiled to a niceness, crisp without but still just faintly pink in the center, spread sparingly with hot mustard, even more sparingly with tart currant jelly and sprinkled with a bit of salt, it's superb fare—to my mind much more flavorful than the ever-same-tasting steak.

And there are these thoughts too:

If your aim is to save cash and cut calories, yet still maintain your reputation as a gourmet cook, consider the less costly cuts of veal. Lean cubes of shoulder of veal can be simmered to glorious Italian ragouts, Hungarian goulashes, and authentic Indian curries, or they can be transformed into that most elegant of French culinary creations, Blanquet de veau, and no one need be even vaguely aware that he is eating low-calorie food. You'll find low-calorie recipes for these dishes in the last chapter of this book, but if your desire is for just a simple hearty, rib-sticking, good-tasting meal—without recipe following—then just substitute veal for beef in your own made-from-memory stew. However, if you are accustomed to browning the meat in oil or shortening, skip this unnecessary step. Instead place veal cubes in a large pot, cover them with water, bring to a full boil. Boil for five minutes, then drain and continue making your stew as it's usually prepared. You'll save money, time and calories by not browning the meat, and it's not necessary to brown veal.

Calorie Cutting with Chicken

There are tricks of the trade here too and they start—as all good cooking starts—with what you buy. For instance, young birds—broilers or fryers—contain less fat than roasting or stewing chickens and are therefore lower in calories. They take less time to cook but can be sub-stituted for the older, tougher birds in any recipe.

Light meat of any age chicken is less calorie-laden than dark meat. Chicken breast is the lowest-calorie part of the bird. Used exclusively for creamed chicken, chicken salad, or stew it makes for grand but low-calorie eating.

But please, oh, please, don't fry either fat or lean chicken or eat it, ever. There are so many better-tasting, easier, less-fattening ways to prepare it. And *don't*, oh, don't, trap all the fat in your chicken by covering it with commercially prepared coating for so-called oven frying. Just read the list of ingredients on the coating package and I'm sure that you won't.

One final *don't*:

When a recipe says words to this effect: "First brown the chicken pieces in oil, butter or other shortening," *don't*. Even lean chicken has ample fat of its own. To brown it perfectly just arrange the pieces of chicken, skin side up, in a single layer in a shallow pan and place the pan in a preheated 375° oven until that side is lightly browned, about 25 minutes. Turn skin side down for about 10 minutes, then turn skin side up again for a final 5 minutes of browning and your chicken is well browned and completely cooked. Drain (see how much fat you are not going to eat?) and proceed, to add the sauce and seasoning of your choice. And continue with your recipe.

Turkey

Portion for portion turkey is even lower in calories than chicken—until you add the stuffing and gravy. But, now, I ask you—did you ever consider roasting and serving a turkey without stuffing and gravy? It can be done and should be done more often. It tastes grand—as does turkey cooked on a rotisserie over glowing coals. For "how to" see recipes in the last chapter of this book.

MORE CALORIE CUTTING WITHOUT CUTTING DOWN ON THE QUANTITY OF FOOD YOU NEED TO APPEASE HUNGER

Dr. Neil Solomon calls the foods listed below zero calorie—which simply means that the number of calories in these foods is just about equal to the amount of energy it makes to chew, digest and absorb them. They have a second bonus too. Rich in nutrients, they also supply bulk and fiber, all of which are necessary to effective weight loss.

Plan your day's diet menu to total up to your allowed calories. Then add any of these vegetables and fruits in any desired variety and amount. Keep in mind, however, that you must include in your basic calorie count any oil, butter or other ingredients used in cooking them or any added to them (such as sugar). Make sure, too, to prepare and cook vegetables so as to retain all nutrients. And eat some raw vegetables as well as raw fruit each day.

FRUITS

Apple
Cantaloupe
Grapefruit
Honeydew
Papaya

Peach
Strawberries
Tangerine
Watermelon

VEGETABLES

Asparagus	Eggplant	Peppers
Bamboo Shoots	Endive	Radishes
Bean Sprouts	Escarole	Rugola
Beets	Fennel	Rutabaga
Broccoli	Green Beans	Rhubarb
Brussels Sprouts	Kale	Spinach
Cabbage	Kohlrabi	Squash
Carrots	Lettuce	Tomatoes
Cauliflower	Mushrooms	Turnips
Celery	Mustard Greens	Turnip Greens
Chard	Okra	Watercress
Chicory	Onions	Wax Beans
Chives	Parsley	
Collard Greens	Pumpkin	

Fish

Creative low-calorie menu planning starts with fish and shellfish. They are low calorie, high protein and loaded with nutrients. I'm for anything that gives you a generous helping of B vitamins, calcium, minerals and polyunsaturated fat, but the fact that I'm mad about fish helps too. Who can get enough Boiled Maine Lobster, Louisiana Shrimp and Oyster Gumbo or Bouillabaisse, the Mediterranean fish stew? They are three of the world's all-time-great dishes. But great too is all fish cookery.

To cut calories drastically, yet eat more and better-tasting food, switch often from meat to fish. Learn to poach it, broil it, bake it and sauce it creatively. You can eat twice as much fish as meat and still come well under your calorie quota.

Fish, too, will free extra calories for the rest of the menu. After an entrée centered around fish, you might want to splurge with a special dessert. Go ahead. You deserve it. Use the recipes for fish preparation that you'll find at the end of this book—they all employ low-calorie cooking methods—but don't stop there. Fish cookery is the most varied and interesting in the world.

Cholesterol and Shellfish

A few years ago shellfish fell from grace. Listed as high-cholesterol foods, they were forbidden on low-fat diets. Well, times and notions change. New discoveries are made and official attitudes are sometimes reversed.

The National Heart and Lung Institute has issued a new edition of its diet manual for the control of cholesterol levels and we're now told that a dieter is probably better off eating lobster or other shellfish than a steak. We are indeed. Consider the facts:

Sirloin steak—3-oz. portion, 475 calories

Crab meat—3-oz. portion, 89 calories

Lobster meat—3-oz. portion, 78 calories

Wow! that's some difference!

A 3-lb. boiled lobster will give you no more than 9 ozs. of meat, but that's a lot of good eating. You can add a big helping of coleslaw and lots of potato straws for a meal that satisfies right down to your toes. You could even start with Clams Casino and end with a wedge of cheesecake and still consider your meal as true diet fare.

Can't afford lobster? No matter. There are literally hundreds of other great diet meals when you plan around fish. See menus in the last chapter.

5

Two Tricks
of the Diet Trade
for Fast, Fast Results

Don't worry too much about calorie counting. Eat all the seafood, fish, chicken, lean meat, vegetables and fruit you desire—but cut out all sugar—not just that teaspoonful that once went into your tea—but any food that contains even a trace of the sweet. Read labels. If sugar is listed as an ingredient, don't buy the product. Unfortunately you'll be surprised at first to find that it's a bit hard to avoid *all* sugar. Today grocer's shelves overflow with sugar-stuffed foods: bread, bouillon, bologna, chili, canned soups, frozen vegetables, mayonnaise, mustard, peanut butter, dips, baked beans and even so-called natural cereals can, and often do, contain sizable amounts of sugar. But it can be bypassed—*if* you are determined—and, with a bit of planning plus judicious buying, you won't miss sugar or what it does to you and your body one bit.

What's wrong with just a bit of sugar if your total diet is calorie low? Nothing really if your body can tolerate it. If you start from zero, then go back to "just a little," you can soon learn how much sugar you personally can eat without disrupting your system and without gaining weight.

Like smog, refined sugar was unknown to man until about two hundred years ago, so the body handles it as a foreign substance. In nature, sugar is packaged with vitamins and minerals. While a potato nets the same glucose as a candy bar, the process differs. Sucrosè (refined sugar) is dumped into the system quickly, but fructose and other naturally occurring sugars, such as lactose in milk and maltose in malt, dribble in and don't shake it up. In addition, refined sugar eludes the appestat, which controls appetite. The body tells you when to stop eating apples but not candy bars.

Refined sugar is so similar to your own blood sugar, which has already been metabolized into glucose, that it escapes processing by your body and goes directly into the intestines as predigested glucose. This throws off the oxygen balance already established in the blood. Fighting to re-establish normal body chemistry, the system gobbles up minerals such as sodium and calcium, which should be used to build and rebuild tissues. Surplus sugar is stored in the liver as glycogen for later use, but if glycogen is in too-great supply, it returns to the blood as fatty acids, which are usually stored in tissues of your stomach, backside and thighs. Residues can be toxic, making you feel sluggish and/or jittery.

To sum up: The body has to use its vitamins, minerals and acids to fight the onrush of refined sugar. This can lower your own blood sugar—which means your body's energy is lower than it was before eating, causing you to be tired, often mentally slow and irritable, plus what's even more to the point here—you have a real desire for more and then more sugar-filled foods for the quick "lift" you think they will give.

Yet that seeming burst of energy from that quick sugar snack or bubbly sugar drink is just the jolt of your system swinging into action to fight the adverse effect on your body and can only leave you even more down and with more excess pounds than ever.

Cut out all sugar for several days, if possible for a full week. Then keep your sugar intake down to size—a little sugar in prepared foods and an occasional, but only very occasional, special sweet treat. The oversweet life can only undermine your health and contribute to your overweight.

But what do you do about your sweet tooth—your very real desire for sweet foods? Your best route is to turn to naturally sweet fruits.

Instead of a cola drink, try unsweetened pineapple juice. It's super sweet mixed half and half with club soda (or, if you can afford it, with imported Perrier water) and poured over plenty of ice cubes in a tall glass. Or—equally sweet—use ripe-watermelon juice. To obtain it, purée seeded cubes of this melon in your electric blender or force them through a sieve. Or try fresh grape juice. Don't use your blender here. Just force big ripe purple grapes through a sieve.

Instead of a Teen-age-Concoction of gooey fudge try (if you simply *must* have a substitute that is equally sweet) this Oriental confection. It's calorie high, but one piece with your dinner coffee will keep you from even more fattening sugar-based desserts.

ORIENTAL SWEETS

¼ lb. seedless raisins
¼ lb. dried figs
½ lb. pitted dates
¼ lb. shelled and blanched almonds
¼ lb. shelled English Walnuts
¼ lb. shelled hickory nuts or pecans
Unsweetened coconut or carob powder

Mix together and put through fine blade of grinder or chop "exceedingly fine." Form into small balls (dip your hands in cold water as you work; the mixture is sticky) and roll in unsweetened coconut or carob power. (Will keep packed in layers between sheets of waxed paper.)

NOTE: Unsweetened coconut is difficult to obtain these days. If you have time and care to take the trouble (it's worth it really), grate fresh coconut, spread out on baking sheet and "dry your own" in a low (200°) oven.

A second confection using unsweetened coconut is childishly easy. Combine 1 cup fresh home-dried coconut with 1 cup (preferably homemade) peanut butter. Shape into small balls and chill until firm.

What are such high-calorie recipes doing in a diet book? Very simple. They are here to convince you that you can indeed live without sugar and without substituting an artificial sweetener, which can't retrain your mind and your appetite away from refined sugar but only keeps you dissatisfied and increases your desire for the so-called real thing.

Other naturally sweet desserts: Purée fresh fruit (peeled and seeded) through a food mill or in a blender. Add a small amount of Cognac or a liqueur if desired. Freeze in ice-cube trays to mushy stage. Pile into parfait glasses and serve "right away."

Dried Fruit: The best kind, from both the standpoint of good sweet taste and super nutrition, are the naturally sun-dried variety. For super-rich treats, stuff jumbo prunes with grated almonds, or dates with walnut halves. For low-calorie, high-nutrition but decidedly "gourmet" non-sugar desserts see Chapter 21.

The cure for alcoholism is a "drying-out period"—total abstinence. So is the treatment for sugarholism. Once you have tried it, you'll feel so much more truly alive, so much more vital, that you will never go back to an oversweet diet again. Which can mean—and it usually does—that you will never consciously need to diet again.

TO SUM UP

Basics of Sugar Avoidance

Switch from soft (sugar) drinks to naturally effervescent mineral water mixed with unsweetened-pineapple or other fresh-fruit juice or drink milk or unsweetened iced tea. Serve crudités as hors d'oeuvres instead of pastries. Snack on fresh or dried fruits instead of candy, and study labels on packaged products for sugar, corn syrup, sucrose or dextrose content.

Ingredients are listed in order of their amount. For example, if sugar is printed second, it means that the product contains more sugar than any other ingredient except the first one listed. You can go one intelligent step further and not buy processed, canned or packaged foods unless they are clearly marked "No sugar added."

"And Season to Taste"

If there were just some "magic" way to lose excess weight . . . There is. Cut down—way down—on salt.

Salt is used entirely too much by many people and its overuse contributes significantly to overweight. Salt tends to retain fluids in the tissues. Many overweight people have a tendency to water retention and an over-salty diet can and does make matters worse.

As a cookbook writer and an avid reader of other peoples' cookbooks, I have found that whenever salt is an ingredient, most authors automatically use "1 teaspoon salt" for almost all recipes intended to serve four to six. Why not ½ tsp. salt? Or, in many cases, why salt at all? It's often not needed, but old habits are strong! When a recipe calls for a specific quantity of salt, don't be a slavish follower. Skip the salt entirely. Weight loss becomes easier when you substitute another seasoning. Try a salt substitute or fresh lemon or lime juice, basil, dillweed, thyme, dried or fresh parsley or fresh garlic. All are good. Like sugar, salt is often more habit than taste.

6
The Great Balancing Act

Just being thin isn't enough. There's no real beauty without good health and for good health you must have a balanced diet, one that contains not only proteins, vitamins and minerals but also carbohydrates and fats in the right proportions. You can cut down on calories but not on nutrients. In fact that's just what you must do for a slim and beautiful body.

Read over the information that follows; develop an awareness of the specific nutrition you can obtain in these foods, then practice a constant balancing act between calories and nutrition each day, not just while you are trying to lose weight but all of your life. This alone will keep you slim and beautiful.

CITRUS FRUITS AND OTHER FRUITS AND VEGETABLES FOR VITAMIN C

Essential for healthy teeth and gums. Builds strong body cells and blood vessels. Not established but strongly believed by a growing number of scientists, doctors, nutritionists and just everyday people with a strong motivation to be and stay healthy: vitamin C aids in the prevention and cure of colds, flu and other related ailments. It's certainly worth trying; there's no beauty in a runny nose.

Vitamin C cannot be stored in the body, so it's extremely important to replenish the supply every day.

Too many people believe that the best way to obtain this vitamin is to drink a glass of orange juice each day, usually the frozen variety mixed with water, but the truth is that frozen or bottled orange juice has probably been robbed of much of its vitamin-C content. Vitamin C is extremely perishable and when orange juice has been exposed to heat and light (almost inevitable in the processed variety) the vitamin-C content is greatly reduced. Also oranges are the highest-calorie citrus fruit. Instead try fresh lemon or lime juice, high in vitamin-C content and lowest in calories of the citrus fruits.

Now, the juice of one lemon in a glass of hot water may be good for you, but ugh! So try this instead: the juice of one lemon or lime in about ¼ cup of (canned) unsweetened pineapple juice. Pour over plenty of ice cubes in a tall glass and fill to the brim with bubbly, sparkly Perrier water (imported French naturally effervescent mineral water). It's a positively exhilarating drink. Champagne without the side effects. And this combination contains more vitamin C than that nursery-school frozen reconstituted orange juice.

There's no law that says you must have vitamin C for breakfast, though most people do enjoy fruit or fruit juice in the morning. The pineapple-lemon-Perrier combination is particularly refreshing first thing out of bed, but there are numerous other low-calorie foods that are super rich in this vitamin to be enjoyed for luncheon or dinner.

Fresh, deep-green parsley, for instance, can add to your vitamin-C intake. Most people waste parsley—simply by not eating it. You know when the recipe reads, "Garnish with parsley and serve." What a really stupid idea! Parsley is too pungent to be eaten this way, so it remains untasted on the plate. It does, however, add immeasurable flavor when it is minced very finely and sprinkled over—not just served with—many types of food: scrambled eggs, creamed chicken, creamed dried chipped beef or tuna fish—all become out of the ordinary when sprinkled lavishly with minced parsley. It's also great in salads, on a baked potato or other vegetable and it decidedly lends an additional dimension to Indian curry or Oriental stir-fry dishes.

Buy your parsley where the merchant has the sense to keep it on ice; it should be crisp not limp, and dark, vivid green in color. Better yet, grow your own. It can even be grown successfully in a sunny kitchen window. I knew a girl in Charleston, South Carolina, who had two window boxes of lush green parsley each spring and it flourished until winter.

Cut as you use it, parsley is high in vitamin content and, as a bonus, it acts as an antitoxic factor in your body. If you eat a generous supply, you will never need to use a deodorant and, moreover, it is mildly diuretic.

Another source of vitamin C is fresh green cabbage. Just make sure you are getting the green crisp variety, not the lifeless white kind that means the outer leaves have wilted and been pulled off. Fresh cabbage finely shredded and mixed with minced green pepper, chopped apple and homemade mayonnaise is positively divine. It also has the added plus of being inexpensive. Or you can steam wedges of cabbage for a perfect accompaniment to a slice of corned beef, or cook it sweet-and-sour style or any number of other ways. In short, it's a highly versatile vegetable that can add variety and interest to the dieter's menu.

Potatoes baked in their skins also supply vitamin C along with other vitamins and minerals. No, they are not fattening when eaten at their best, plain without the usual unnecessary embellishments of cream, butter and such. A dash of salt, a sprinkling of freshly ground pepper and perhaps a little minced parsley are all a good baked potato needs. For variety try stuffing them with cottage and Parmesan cheese. You'll find the recipe on page 95. Just be sure to eat the skin too; it's rich in vitamins and minerals.

Fresh ripe tomatoes—preferably home grown, or at least grown locally and vine-ripened, then sliced thin and marinated in a simple homemade French dressing—offer another great and delicious way to add to your vitamin-C quota.

Other good sources, fresh strawberries and cantaloupe which, combined, make an elegant fruit compote. Add a judicious bit of any good liqueur and it's party fare. Par excellence also, when obtainable, are exotic mangoes and papayas. The list is long, all mouth-watering and there's this bonus—almost all vitamin-C-rich foods pass the low-calorie test. This is important because you need all you can eat and still stay within your calorie quota, particularly if you smoke, or drink even a small amount of hard liquor, both of which deplete your body of vitamin C.

LEAFY DARK GREEN AND YELLOW VEGETABLES FOR VITAMIN A

When you think vitamin A, think color and think what it can do for you. It's essential for healthy blemish-free skin, clear eyes and lustrous hair. Essential too for good vision. Without it, you will soon develop frown lines and squinty eyes.

Your body makes its own vitamin A from foods containing carotene—leafy green vegetables, which also offer an added benefit in that they are also rich in iron and vitamin C.

Learn to cook Southern-style collard greens, mustard and turnip greens—and drink the "pot liquor" (the cooking liquid) too. These are grand eating and can make a Confederate out of any Yankee who will give them a fair try. However, if you remain unconvinced, spinach also provides ample vitamin A in the diet as does broccoli, and the green outer leaves of lettuce. Another do-gooder if you will eat it, not just look at it on your plate, is watercress.

Also rich in vitamin A are the deep yellow vegetables. Tender young carrots, for instance. Try your best to get the kind that still has leafy green tops, a sure sign that they are not the storage variety. Sweet potatoes are a particularly rich source and, no, they are not fattening. Yellow squash, both the summer and winter variety, also contain an ample supply of vitamin A, as do pumpkins and tomatoes.

Needed each day for an ample supply of vitamin A are one or more servings of the above vegetables raw or cooked, such as a small baked sweet potato, a half cantaloupe or a salad made from crisp outer green leaves of lettuce (the Boston variety is preferable to the iceberg type) combined with parsley and, if possible, watercress. Vitamin A is not easily destroyed by cooking, so if you substitute or add a serving of steamed carrots, yellow squash or the baked sweet potato in place of raw vegetable or fruit, you will still be getting a good part of your vitamin A quota.

OTHER ESSENTIAL FRUITS AND VEGETABLES FOR A TOTAL BALANCE OF VITAMINS AND MINERALS

The foods in this group are not super rich in any one vitamin such as C or A, but eaten along with the above two groups they can total up to generous quantities of essential nutrients that will not only keep you healthy but can help you lose weight.

Choose from bananas, pineapple, apples, peaches, plums, et cetera.

Vegetable choices include beets, turnips, artichokes, Brussels sprouts, eggplant, celery, cucumbers, et cetera.

Eaten raw, "out of hand" or nicely sliced on a plate, fresh fruit can help speed up your digestion and thus help burn up or assimilate fats and carbohydrates and, of course, calories; as can many raw or briefly cooked vegetables. Have you ever tried peeled and thinly sliced turnips (dip them in a lemony ice water bath to retard darkening) as a base for creamy soft cheddar cheese? Or any other cheese or meat spread for that matter. They are crisp and delicious, much better than any so-called cocktail cracker.

Very young flowerets of broccoli are great for dunking, as are stalks of green celery and cucumber slices—all weightless wonders to replace the calorie-high snack.

RECOMMENDED SERVINGS

Generally four small servings a day—two of vegetables, two of fruit—are recommended on a calorie-restricted diet, but I say eat all the fresh, tender vegetables and ripe, juicy fruit that you can find at your market or grow in your garden. They are health insurance and will help you to lose weight by cutting your appetite for high-calorie food.

FISH AND SHELLFISH, POULTRY AND MEATS

To be sure of getting a good supply of many different nutrients as well as protein, choose a wide variety from the group below, but to keep calories low give preference as listed. Think first of fish and shellfish, then of poultry and finally of meat.

All too many people think only of red meat, or more specifically beef, when they think of protein and therefore conclude that all protein is expensive. But just a little research can prove that this is far from true. Actually beef is a poor protein buy for the dieter because it's expensive in calorie cost too. A 3-oz. piece of sirloin steak supplies 20 grams of protein but weighs in at 330 calories, while 3 ozs. of lean broiled chicken will give you the same protein count for about half the calories. So will 3 ozs. of canned sardines.

To get the most protein for the lowest calorie investment at the least cost consider the list below. Each food has extra qualities that add to its nutritional (as well as beauty and health-giving) values:

3 ozs. calves liver, about 120 calories for each 15 grams protein

3 ozs. sardines (canned), about 175 calories for about 20 grams protein

3 ozs. shrimp, about 100 calories for about 21 grams protein

3 ozs. crabmeat, about 85 calories for about 15 grams protein

3 ozs. (canned) tuna, about 170 calories for about 24 grams protein

3 ozs. fish fillets (non-oily type), about 133 calories for 22 grams protein

3 ozs. (canned) salmon, about 120 calories for about 17 grams protein

2 ozs. dried chipped beef, about 115 calories for about 19 grams protein

3 ozs. broiled chicken, about 115 calories for about 20 grams protein

3 ozs. roasted turkey, about 95 calories for about 14 grams protein
3 ozs. lamb chops, about 14 calories for about 21 grams protein
3 ozs. corned beef, about 185 calories for about 22 grams protein
4 ozs. cottage cheese (uncreamed), about 85 calories for about 17 grams protein

You should have 1 gram of protein every day for every 2 pounds you weigh, or so say the experts. I think a bit more won't hurt you. Get it from any of the inexpensive sources above. The protein you eat is more than just food to keep you going. It's real beauty food for your entire body.

MILK AND MILK FOODS FOR CALCIUM
ALSO FOR PROTEIN AND VITAMINS PLUS

If you don't like skimmed milk (who really does?) and you can't fit whole milk into your calorie allowance, eat tart and tangy, cool and smooth yogurt. It's the only food I know of that not only tastes grand but is non-fattening, inexpensive, legal and good for you too.

Eight ounces of yogurt contain calcium and B vitamins galore, as well as top-quality complete proteins plus riboflavin and phosphorus—all set to work synergistically inside you.

Cook with a tablespoon of plain yogurt and you add only 8 calories, versus 25 for the same amount of sour cream or 65 for mayonnaise.

When making soups, sauces, "creamed" vegetables or mashed potatoes, I reach for yogurt instead of cream, which now seems too rich, clogging and indigestible.

When a recipe calls for cream cheese or ricotta,

substitute cheese made at home from yogurt (see page 214) and you'll find that the flavor is infinitely better.

Yogurt is a natural for "today cooks" who want lighter, but better-tasting, low-calorie dishes: at 130 to 150 calories per 8-oz. carton, depending on what brand, yogurt (which currently is selling at 35¢ in my area) has slightly fewer calories than whole milk—but you can eat less and get more nutrition. When compared to other dairy products, the difference between calorie count and cost seems astronomical. Just read this: 8 ozs. of the following—half and half, 332 calories, 35¢; sour cream, 485 calories, 35¢; light cream, 506 calories, 45¢; heavy cream, 832 calories, 79¢. You can see why both eating yogurt and cooking with it is one of the simplest, easiest, most delicious and satisfactory ways to cut calorie intake *and* cost.

Yogurt has this plus too. It has the seemingly magical ability to smooth and blend flavors like curry powder, chili powder and mustard, making them more subtle and mellow.

You can blend yogurt into clear, fat-free beef stock for a fabulous "cream" gravy. You can whirl it in a blender with frozen fruit to make a dessert sauce for fresh fruit. You can use it instead of milk to make light low-calorie "buttermilk" biscuits. Mix it; half and half, with home-made mayonnaise for an ambrosia-like salad dressing, and use it as a suitable and satisfactory substitute in almost all recipes instead of sour cream. In fact it's the "everything" ingredient for all light-minded cooks.

WHOLE GRAIN FOR B VITAMINS AND IRON, CARBOHYDRATES AND SOME PROTEIN

Tops on the list is wheat germ, with all the beauty vitamins and minerals. There is more nutrition in a tablespoon of wheat germ than in a loaf of many of our so-called enriched breads. For a truly nourishing bread, make your own from stone-ground flour with wheat germ added. But watch it—bread, especially nourishing bread, is calorie high. If you serve any bread at a meal, serve it instead of—not with—rice, potatoes or other such food. And make sure it is a bread "so good" it can be eaten with pleasure sans butter or other high-calorie spread. All sandwiches on dieters' menus are "open face": plenty of filling but only one slice of bread.

Make your own whole-grain cereals. Ingredients are available at any good health-food store. Most commercially prepared packaged whole-grain cereals are loaded with sugar. If you do buy them, read the label first.

FATS AND OILS TO MAKE USE OF VITAMINS A AND E, HANDLE CHOLESTEROL, BURN FOODS FOR ENERGY AND NOURISH THE SKIN

Don't make the mistake of cutting all fats from your diet. It won't work. Your skin and hair will reflect it in a dull, dingy, flaky look if you attempt a fat-free diet.

But learn to separate the bad from the good and cut out the former.

You don't need—and will undoubtedly live longer, healthier and slimmer without—lard, processed cheese and animal fat. You can use with good results: avocado oil, corn oil, peanut oil, safflower oil, sunflower oil, soy oil and wheat-germ oil. All are good for you and are polyunsaturated, which means, technically, "rich in unsaturated chemical bonds." These oils do not combine in the blood stream to form fatty deposits on the walls of the arteries. Any oil you use for cooking should be polyunsaturated.

EGGS AND CHEESE FOR LOW-CALORIE PROTEIN PLUS SOME VERY VALUABLE NUTRIENTS

Nothing satisfies the appetite as quickly as a hard-cooked egg and nothing could taste better than such an egg halved, spread with Dijon mustard and topped with a slice of crisp pickle.

Although eggs do contain some cholesterol, they are a rich source of lecithin, which helps the body utilize cholesterol normally—canceling out the idea that they should be eaten only occasionally if at all.

Eggs and cheese supply low-calorie protein with an abundance of amino acids essential to health. In addition eggs supply some iron plus vitamin A and B_2. Cheese furnishes some calcium and B_2 as well.

Skip processed cheeses—they are all made solid largely by the hydrogenation of the butter fat and that you don't need—but make natural cheese and eggs a part of your diet plan. Both can help you lose weight and gain beauty and health.

Semisoft cheeses are lower in calories than the hard variety. Lowest of all is cottage cheese, one of the dieter's best friends. But a word of warning here: Cottage cheese can become an enemy and turn on you. If eaten plain and served every day, you may find it so boring that you'll slide off the diet wagon because of a longing for "something that tastes really good"—like a slice of chocolate cake "just this once."

Cottage cheese is great low-calorie fare, but it should seldom, if ever, be served "as is." It should be used instead as a "base" ingredient. Mix it with a goodly amount of minced celery, cucumber and tart apple, season with a bit of Tabasco plus a little salt and freshly ground black pepper and serve as a dip. Or serve it, mixed with a bit of whipped butter and honey, for your morning toast. Or make it into a delicious and sinfully rich-tasting ice cream (see recipe page 222), but serve it plain only at your own risk.

7
Water!

If you want it "all"—beauty, a slim body, energy and an alert mind—then, right now, today, become a dropout from the poopsi generation and give up "the real thing." It cannot "add life," as currently advertised, only excess pounds. It took courage to write those words. They sound so un-American, but, before I'm deported or this book is banned as subversive, hear me out.

Do you really believe that those marvelous, vitally alive young people you see on the TV screen, joyously cycling through the park or gleefully plunging into the pounding surf, actually drink the stuff? Let me assure you that very few of them do. It takes stamina and self-discipline to stay on top in commercial television and these kids remain there, not by imbibing carbonated sugar drinks, but by paying strict attention to what they do—and do not—eat and drink to maintain their good looks, slim bodies and great health. They are aware of the fact that "soft" drinks are hard on the figure and do not, as is implied, quench thirst.

For thirst quenching they drink what really is "the real thing"—zero-calorie water.

Either plain, or not so plain, water is one of the best aids to weight control you can find at any price—and there's this bonus too: Water can help you have clear, unblemished, wrinkle-free skin. Dr. Ernst Lazlo, who was one of the world's most renowned dermatologists, once said, "If there wasn't any water, I would have had to invent it."

Used internally and externally water is basic in your fight against overweight.

Nicole Ronsard in her book on cellulite (which is just another name for stubborn, hard-to-lose fat) advises eight glasses of water a day to cleanse the body of wastes and residues. This may be a bit much for a non-water drinker to tolerate at the beginning, but she is right. A high-protein, low-salt, lots-of-water diet will result in loss of weight. It can't help but do so. One or two glasses of water about an hour before a meal will cut your appetite down to size. You can't overeat. You simply won't want all that food.

But that's only part of the water story.

Many would-be gourmets, after a vacation in France, are surprised to find on return that for some miraculous reason they did not gain weight even though they had eaten, to say it politely, luxuriously, without a calorie thought. I strongly suspect that the bottled mineral water they "discovered" on so many French restaurant tables helped to counteract their indulgences. Though there is no medical basis of fact in this theory, I've seen it happen time and again. Like apple cider vinegar the mineral water seems to be a factor in stabilizing weight.

We Americans are just beginning to learn about water and we have a lot more to learn.

The first thing to be aware of concerning water is so simple that it seems obvious, but a lot of people forget it: If you are going to use ordinary tap water, let it run several minutes before filling your glass; the water in the pipes is stale and simply doesn't taste as good. This holds true for water used in cooking as well. Your coffee or tea will taste a lot better if you start with cold fresh water; hot water should be used only for your shower or bath.

Actually, if you are serious about losing weight, you should cultivate a taste for bottled mineral water. It not only tastes delicious but, as I have mentioned, can actually cut down your appetite. The following is a list of mineral waters I have found both helpful and pleasurable:

Mountain Valley Water
This is the water De Soto found the Indians drinking when he discovered Hot Springs, Arkansas, in 1541. One of the best, and mildly diuretic, it has a cool, refreshing taste and, not incidentally, makes the best coffee and tea that I have ever had. Diana Vreeland, one of the top fashion experts of all time, never fails to have a bottle of Mountain Valley on her desk and she is as famed for her vital young figure as she is for her fashion expertise.

Evian Water
From the springs at Evian-les-Bains in the French Alps. This is the best-selling bottled water in the world. In France it is the classic cure for just about anything.

Fiuggi
From Italy, not as well known as the first two, but I am told Michelangelo claimed it dissolved his kidney stones.

Perrier
My all-time favorite, naturally effervescent and simply delicious. From the springs near Marseilles in France. Over 400 million of the familiar green bottles are shipped all over the world every year.

There are, of course, other bottled waters, but these are generally available and each is wonderful in its own way. I think you will find that Perrier water combined with fruit juice makes a highly refreshing substitute for calorie-high soft drinks. Try half fresh orange or half pineapple juice and half Perrier water and I'll guarantee you will never go back to colas. A glass of mineral water with plenty of ice and a slice of lemon makes a calorie-free substitute for the cocktail hour too.

While on the subject of what to drink, properly made tea and coffee can be a big help toward losing weight. A cup of really good hot tea made with fresh boiling water, using 1 teaspoon of tea for each cup, then served with a slice of lemon has great "pick up" quality. Try it midmorning and afternoon as a substitute for that morning Danish or the afternoon cola drink. Once you get the habit, you'll never go back to junky snacks.

As for coffee, if you are presently using cream and sugar, it's probably because the coffee tastes pretty terrible. Learn how to make really perfect coffee and you will actually prefer it black.

The first step toward making perfect coffee is your selection of a coffeepot, and the only type that will give you a clear, fresh-tasting, fragrant brew is one that uses a filter paper. Most people don't realize it, but coffee contains oil that is released upon contact with hot water and it is this oil that makes for bitter coffee. When the oil is trapped by a filter, the result is clear, delicious coffee that can even be reheated. Instead of using boiling water when you make coffee, use water which is barely simmering—the lower temperature causes less oil to be released. If you really want perfect coffee, buy it in the bean and grind only what you need for one pot. If this sounds like a lot of trouble and expense, it isn't. Small grinders are to be had for about ten dollars and A & P Bokar-brand bean coffee is available across the country. You will use less coffee too as it is fresher and therefore stronger and that's no small consideration.

I am sure at this point you will regard me as a coffee

nut, but I have found a good cup of coffee a great help in weight loss. If you are one of those people who have to have something to "go with" your coffee, put a teaspoon of Cognac (or brandy) in it and I assure you that you will enjoy your "coffee break" solo as much as you did with the snacky food or cream and sugar that you once used to accompany every cup.

One last point about coffee: Store it in the freezer—whether the bean or ground variety. This is particularly important with ground coffee as exposure to light and heat will turn the best coffee rancid and that also makes for a bitter brew. Now, I'm going to add one thing that will probably annoy a lot of people, but I can't help it: Don't bother with instant coffee. It simply doesn't taste good and you will be tempted to go back to the old cream-and-sugar routine.

But let's get back to tea. Being a Louisiana girl myself, I've always been primarily a coffee drinker, but in recent years I've discovered tea. I must confess to being lazy enough to use tea bags sometimes, but, to tell the truth, since I've had the pleasure of drinking a really good cup of tea, I don't begrudge the few pennies extra and the few moments it takes to make it perfect. Richard Twining organized the Twining Tea Company in the eighteenth century and they still import a variety of quality teas. Experiment with a few until you find your favorite. My personal choice is English breakfast tea, pungent but not too strong. I find a cup or two in the afternoon cuts my appetite and still provides that "little something" most people want toward the end of the day.

Needless to say both tea and coffee are directly related to the water that is used. If you find your tap water unpalatable, spend a few extra pennies and use bottled water. Mountain Valley water is particularly good and makes for really fabulous tea or coffee. If this sounds like an extravagance, stop and think how much you have been spending on cookies, Danish, pies and cakes—no small amount. The water is cheaper and can help you win the battle of the bulge.

Finally don't be afraid of being waterlogged. Water will not stay stored in your body if you eat a high-protein diet; it will simply cleanse you of toxic waste. Mineral water, particularly Mountain Valley, is actually mildly diuretic, not enough to be harmful but enough to keep the motor going. Train yourself to get in those eight glasses a day and you will reap the pleasures of a slim, trim you and a clear, wrinkle-free skin at the same time.

8
A Bonus of Beauty

Losing weight should be only part of your self-improvement plan. Put together an effective weight-loss diet plus some new "beauty habits" and the result is a new you.

First things first. The basics of a sound, healthy body start with a regular checkup with your doctor and a semiannual trip to the dentist. You can't be good-looking with bad teeth.

Now, get yourself on a schedule. Start with a diary to record your weight loss. It will encourage you to keep up the good work. The next thing is to set up a daily program to create a better-looking you. Do you hate to exercise? Well, you won't if you don't make a Federal case out of it. Try five minutes of simply stretching and bending every morning when you first wake up. Follow with a quick shower and a solid tooth-brushing session.

To make sure you are getting enough vitamin C, it helps to have the juice of one lemon in a glass of mineral water before breakfast. Add pineapple juice to it if you like. There's that water theory again, but it does work.

At night a warm bath can soothe jangled nerves as effectively as the before-dinner cocktail and it's a lot better for the figure. Try a handful of baking soda in the water. It is a great skin soother.

But baking soda is not the only effective beauty maker from your kitchen. Before the current proliferation of commercial cosmetics our grandmothers used natural foods as cosmetics, and they are still highly effective, in fact more so than most of the brand-name variety. Here is a list of them and suggestions for using them:

BEAUTY FOODS

Avocados
Not only a powerhouse of vitamins, minerals and unsaturated oils and a potent help to the dieter, but, rich in vitamin E, they make a highly effective mask for the skin. Vitamin-E oil is one of the few oils that will penetrate the skin. Purée half of a ripe avocado and spread it over your face and neck. (Use a shower cap to keep your hair out of the way.) Leave the mask on while you relax in your bath. Thirty minutes if possible. Your skin will look softer and smoother, particularly if you follow a regular masking schedule. Once a week is preferable. No beauty regimen will work unless it is followed consistently.

Eggs
Much maligned in recent years as a cause for high cholesterol, the egg has come back into respectability. New research has proved that the egg simply isn't guilty. Eggs are an invaluable aid to weight loss. For example, a hard-boiled egg can be a great appetite appeaser and stuffed with a little imagination (see recipe page 179) makes a delicious lunch. But there's more to eggs than eating them. An egg-white mask is highly effective in tightening and firming the skin. It also rids the pores of impurities and leaves your face feeling fresh and clean.

It's simple and inexpensive. Just beat one egg white to a froth, spread it on face and neck and allow it to dry for 15 to 20 minutes. As with the avocado mask, it's a good idea to do this while you have your evening bath. Rinse the mask off with warm water and spread a little plain old vaseline around your eyes, mouth and forehead. It's as effective as the most expensive face cream.

Lemons

Super beauty food both internally and externally. One of the best sources of vitamin C, the juice of one lemon will provide a large measure of your daily requirement of this important vitamin. In addition to helping prevent colds and other infectious diseases, lemon juice and other citrus fruits help to cleanse the body of waste. You will never need a laxative (and certainly you shouldn't take them) if you adopt the habit of drinking a generous glass of grapefruit juice every day plus the lemon juice and mineral water previously mentioned.

As an external beauty aid, lemons can be your secret weapon for beautiful, smooth hands and feet. A half lemon rubbed on cuticles and on rough heels or elbows has a terrific softening effect. It also bleaches out stains and leaves your nails clean and blemish free.

The juice of one lemon, used in warm water as a final rinse for your shampoo, rids your hair of excess oil and adds sheen and body. Lemon juice can also effectively bleach out a yellowing suntan or that awful red-neck look. It is a safe and gentle bleach that can be used as often as you like.

Oatmeal

My all-time favorite food cosmetic. An oatmeal scrub can rid your face and body of dry dead cells, leaving your skin soft and clear. It is particularly effective for blemished skin and will help to eliminate blackheads and clogged pores. For best results, dip into a warm tub of water, then vigorously scrub yourself with oatmeal, using a washcloth or a loofah mat. Rinse off with tepid water and rub yourself dry with a terry towel. Follow with hand cream and your whole body will feel silky smooth.

Honey

One of nature's most valuable gifts. Used in place of refined sugar, it can be a delicious and easy way to add valuable nutrition to anyone's diet. Once you try honey as a sugar substitute, I doubt if you will ever change. There are any number of honeys to choose from and it's fun to experiment, but just be sure you get natural raw honey. It not only tastes better than honey that has been processed by heat treatment, but it's better for you.

Honey is also invaluable for the skin. A honey mask will firm and tighten facial skin. Spread it on lightly and leave it while you have your bath. Rinse off with warm water followed by a splash of cold. A program of "kitchen aids," followed consistently, will lead to a clearer more beautiful skin, stronger better-looking fingernails and, most important, a new pride in the way you look, which is perhaps the most essential factor in keeping you on a sane, healthful pattern of eating.

The important thing is not to regard time spent on yourself as time wasted. You are important and you cannot function effectively as a person useful to yourself and to others without feeling and looking your best. Vital, healthy human beings can contribute much to life for themselves and others. Half-well people, disappointed in themselves, cannot. It's as simple as that. Time and effort devoted to becoming—and staying—supremely fit is well spent, not only for yourself but for all of the people in your life—family, friends, fellow workers, anyone with whom you come in contact. Think about it. Wouldn't you rather be around a cheerful, attractive, healthy person? Most people would, so you are doing the world a favor when you care for yourself.

THE BEAUTIFUL-PERSON CHART

Make out a schedule for yourself. Only you can do it, for only you know what your responsibilities and chores may be. What's right for the woman who has children and a house to care for can be all wrong for the man or girl with a job. There are, however, certain things you should do for yourself every day, every week and every year. Make up your own schedule from the following list. How you fit it into your own life is not important. What is important is that you *do* fit it in for maximum health and beauty and that, of course, includes a slim, trim body.

YEARLY: A thorough medical checkup.

SEMIANNUALLY: Dentist appointment for checkup and cleaning.

MONTHLY: Hair and scalp treatment; hair cut or trim; color if you use it.

Wardrobe check for cleaning, repairs or replacement.

WEEKLY: Shampoo and hair set, manicure.

Facial mask.

Take your measurements too.

DAILY: Brisk, cold shower.

Twice daily (at least)—thorough tooth-brushing.

Weight check for progress.

Minimum of 15 minutes exercise, preferably 30. Can include a brisk walk.

Hot, relaxing bath.

Thorough face and neck cleansing.

Massage of feet, hands and elbows with creamy lotion.

BLENDER DRINKS FOR FAST PICKUP MAY BE SUBSTITUTED FOR YOUR USUAL BREAKFAST OR EVEN LUNCH

A blender is a great help in cutting calories and stepping up nutrition. Try these combinations and then you'll probably make up a few of your own:

1 cup milk
5 or 6 dried apricots
1 tbs. wheat germ

1 cup milk
1 small banana
½ cup orange juice

1 cup milk
5 or 6 cooked and pitted prunes
½ cup yogurt

1 cup milk
1 cup peeled and sliced fresh peaches
1 tbs. wheat germ

1 cup orange juice
1 cup unsweetened pineapple juice
½ cup yogurt

1 cup milk
½ cup apple juice
1 peeled and sliced fresh apple

1 cup milk
1 cup washed and hulled strawberries
1 tbs. wheat germ

All combinations are for one serving and of course the preparation is simplicity itself. Just combine the various ingredients in a blender and whirl to a froth at high speed.

9
Menu-planning for a Twenty-first-Century Diet

To lose weight without regimented dieting, become familiar with the approximate calorie count of all of the food that you eat—one small inexpensive book listing the calorie values of most food will keep you informed—but don't be a slave to calorie counting. It is only necessary for you to be sufficiently knowledgeable to plan a balanced menu that will achieve a total low-calorie meal. For example, if you plan on serving fish with a really great but high-calorie sauce and steamed new potatoes, you can bring the total calorie count down by selecting a vegetable so calorie low that the total count of the meal will fit into your daily calorie allowance.

When menu-planning, think first of fish or shellfish. They are always lower in calories than meat. Next choice, turkey or chicken, both lower in calories than most meats. However, if meat is your choice, think first of glandular meats, such as kidneys or liver. Either one is a powerhouse of nutrients, calorie low in comparison to beef, pork or lamb, yet just as high, or higher, in appetite satisfaction.

Serve meat less often and when you do serve it, serve less than usual portions. Three-quarters of a pound of ground meat will make four hamburger patties almost as big as one pound of meat. You can serve two people steaks with 1 lb. of beef, or you can use ½ lb. of beef to serve four if it's prepared with low-calorie vegetables in an Oriental stir-fry dish or as part of a hearty and satisfying old-fashioned stew.

Before you think about potatoes, rice or bread as an accompaniment to meat, think of fresh vegetables. Yes, there is always something fresh in the market. Why fresh instead of frozen or canned? Because fresh vegetables not only give you the most nutrients for the least calories, but also the most flavor, appetite satisfaction and enjoyment. All frozen vegetables have been blanched—partially cooked—before being frozen. Thus they are robbed of a good part of their nutrients as well as much of their flavor. Canned vegetables have undergone a similar heating process. Two vegetables are just as satisfying as a starch and one vegetable.

Make fresh fruit a daily part of your diet—not just as a between-meal appetite appeaser, though it is one of the best—but as part of a meal. A broiled fresh peach half can make special an otherwise dull broiled-lamb-chop-and-baked-potato meal. Baked bananas add richness to roast chicken, and grapefruit sections are an elegant "go with" for poached fish.

If you are going to serve bread, skip the rice or potatoes. In other words, serve only one starchy food with a meal.

Skip dessert? It's not necessary. Just make it a low-sugar, low-calorie fruit compote, or fruit ice or gelatin made with fresh fruit.

Don't make dieting a punishment for your sin of overweight. Dry toast and a poached egg are a pretty sad alternate to hot biscuits, butter and jam, but if you substitute a ripe peach, a wedge of mellow Camembert and whole-wheat wafers with your coffee, you won't miss the biscuits one bit. Or if, instead of a salad of cottage cheese and water-packed peaches at the corner drugstore, you order an antipasto with a glass of red wine at the best Italian restaurant in town, you're not dieting—just having a great meal.

AND FINALLY SWEEP AWAY SOME OF THOSE MYTHS ABOUT DIETING

Myth 1: You must eat three meals a day to diet successfully yet retain your health.

Refutation: Not necessarily. So, as long as your weekly calorie intake does not exceed your weekly calorie expenditure, you can budget your calories to suit your life-style. Skipping an occasional meal can help you lose weight—as can one day of fasting—though more can put you below your necessary nutritional needs.

Myth 2: Eating a well-rounded breakfast can help you remain on a diet for the balance of the day.

Refutation: That depends on what you call a well-rounded breakfast. Eggs and bacon and grits and biscuits it's not. A well-balanced breakfast can be a fruit shake made in seconds in your electric blender—a handful of strawberries, a glass of skimmed milk, a little wheat germ, some dry skimmed-milk powder, and one raw egg—that's a powerhouse breakfast that will keep you going without hunger until late in the day. But so will a whole orange, plus a slice of panbroiled liver with a bit of Worcestershire sauce, served on a slice of whole-grain "health-loaf" bread and a cup of black coffee. Or yogurt over sliced bananas, sprinkled with wheat germ and unsweetened tea. Or nothing at all until noon—some people simply are not hungry early in the day.

Myth 3: Eating before you go to bed puts on pounds.

Refutation: When you eat has nothing to do with

weight gain. Calories do. You gain weight only when the number of calories consumed during the day exceeds the total number of calories expended during the day. If you are a night person and like to eat late, enjoy it. It's your right.

Myth 4: *Dieting without going hungry just isn't possible.*

Refutation: Not so, not so, although it is true that bad eating habits must be changed for good ones. You can't expect to lose weight with Danish and coffee for breakfast; jelly donuts midmorning; a hamburger with French fries, apple pie and a cola drink for lunch, followed by a dinner of fried fish and more fried potatoes—but you can select low-calorie foods that are both appetizing and sufficiently filling so that you need never feel deprived.

A high-protein breakfast, featuring a small broiled steak or a slice of calves liver, will cut your desire for a midmorning snack. So will a blender milk shake made with skimmed milk, fresh fruit (especially bananas), a teaspoon or so of brewer's yeast, with a bit of honey and a dash of cinnamon to mask the yeast taste.

Yogurt over fresh fruit for lunch may not be as emotionally satisfying as a hamburger, but it will be even more filling—for about one-quarter the calories. So will a more glamorous luncheon menu of cold shrimp in vinaigrette sauce, a wedge of semi-soft cheese, a ripe pear and black coffee; or a chef's salad topped with strips of Swiss cheese and turkey plus wedges of hard-cooked egg and one or two green olives for both flavor and color. Such high-protein fare will dull your appetite and eliminate your desire for a midafternoon sweet.

As for dinner, you can again be filled, and luxuriously so, by a careful choice of low-calorie, high-protein food. There is no excuse for hunger pangs when you know how to select, cook and enjoy such food.

Myth 5: *It doesn't matter what you eat as long as you*

eat fewer calories than your body needs to maintain its present weight.

Refutation: This final myth contains some measure of truth, but along with your weight loss you may lose both your beauty and your health. Most foods on today's market are so over-processed and refined, so loaded with additives and preservatives, that they are robbed of most of their original nutritional properties. This is the case with most so-called convenience foods, which have low nutritional value and offer little else but starch and calories. It's harder to lose weight with such foods and what's convenient about that? A wedge of cheese and an apple, plus a small glass of red wine is more convenient. The protein-rich cheese will satisfy your appetite much more easily than a frozen chicken pie and the apple, with its natural fiber, can actually speed up your weight loss.

Creative Low-Calorie Cooking

Just what is creative low-calorie cooking? Simply this: enjoying menus that are interesting and flavorful enough to keep you on a low-calorie regimen. Happily there are numerous ways to trick your appetite into being satisfied without high-calorie foods. Suggested here are only a few of the ideas that you will find put to use in the menus and recipes to follow in the next chapter.

Use stock (see pages 127-31) both beef and chicken. Nothing will add more flavor and nutrition to low-calorie dishes than well-made stock. For a truly Epicurean experience try the recipe for low-calorie Ris de Veau Marchand du Vin (see pages 171-72) (sweetbreads in wine sauce) or the Indian Curry (see pages 150-51) thickened not with flour and cream but with rich, flavorful chicken stock and puréed apples. Both are low calorie but high in appetite satisfaction, the kind of food you look forward to, not a dreary dieter's lamb chop with a serving of steamed spinach.

Next in importance to your ever-present supply of stock is the imaginative use of seasoning. The calorie count is nil in freshly ground black Java pepper and it is well worth the small amount of time and money invested. A plain poached or boiled egg for breakfast takes on flavor plus when sprinkled with a trace of salt, fresh pepper and a bit of minced parsley.

Tabasco, the hot red-pepper sauce from Louisiana, can add immeasurably to soups, stews, sauces and even scrambled eggs. It will also step up ordinary cocktail sauce, turning a shrimp cocktail into a high-powered, protein-rich lunch when served with a quarter of hard-boiled egg and a piece of Melba toast. To say that the calorie count is low is an understatement.

Lemons: both the juice and the grated peel are wonderful seasoning. A wedge of lemon squeezed over broiled fish or oysters adds a real flavor bonus. You won't find broiled fish a dull uninspiring dish if you zip up the flavor with Tabasco, lemon juice and black pepper. That fresh lemon is a must for a gourmet's plate of iron-rich, very low-calorie, raw oysters is almost too obvious to mention. Grated rind will add zest and interest to a compote of fresh fruit. Sweeten the compote with honey and add a tablespoon or so of Cognac or liqueur such as Grand Marnier and you will never miss the gooey slice of cake or the calorie-laden piece of pie.

To add the spice of life to a dieter's menu, try baking an apple with honey as a sweetener and a sprinkling of cinnamon. Serve with a dollop of yogurt for a super dessert or even as a great breakfast. Apple Betty made with wheat germ, honey and cinnamon is mighty good too.

Basil, preferably fresh (grow a pot of it in your kitchen window), transforms a broiled tomato from so-so to superb.

Learn to experiment with spices. Many recipes in this

book use such powerhouse seasoning magic as sesame and mustard seed, coriander, ginger and mixed Italian herbs.

All add great flavor—and almost zero calories—to any number of dishes.

One word of advice, however—keep dried spices *and* pepper in the refrigerator. Those charming (?) spice racks you see hung over a stove are death to freshness and flavor.

Wine is an essential flavoring in diet cookery. A necessity in making stock (the acid brings out the natural gelatin of the bones), it also adds immeasurable flavor. No, it does not add calories. The alcohol content—and thus the calories—evaporate during the cooking process and only the flavor remains.

Wine is a great flavor asset in many sauces, soups and desserts. Try poaching oranges or pears in red wine for a low-calorie but super-tasting finish to a meal. A bit of sherry added to soup can transform an otherwise dull luncheon of clear beef broth and crackers. There's no harm either in a glass of chilled white wine with broiled chicken for dinner.

Wine adds flavor even to vegetable dishes. The spinach recipe (on p. 191) uses Madeira to change this usually dull, but good-for-you, vegetable into a "special."

COGNAC AND LIQUEURS

Here's the magic touch that adds supreme flavor to just about everything from soup to dessert. Ordinary (very lean) ground beef is transformed by browning the patties, then flaming them with Cognac or brandy. (This also burns up surface fat.) Add a bit of beef stock and a small amount of red wine and cook briefly in the sauce. Serve hot over a thin piece of toast, accompanied by the pan juice. Or try chicken, oven-browned, fat poured off, and then flamed with Cognac on top of the stove. Add chicken stock, white wine, and mushrooms. Cook, covered, until chicken is tender. You won't be bored with this kind of dish.

Cognac, egg yolks, cream and sugar makes a superb and seemingly sinfully rich sauce for fruit (see recipe page 220), but only a teaspoon or two over fresh fruit, particularly low-calorie strawberries. It seems a real indulgence and when served so sparingly it cuts out your desire for more fattening desserts. It will keep for several days in the refrigerator, to use for a dessert touch to any fruit for at least a week.

Any liqueur—kirsch and Grand Marnier in particular—transforms fruit compotes. And try a broiled grapefruit half sweetened with a little honey, then sprinkled with kirsch. It just might become your favorite dessert.

Mustard, catsup, chili sauce and steak sauce, though they contain a few calories, can, when used sparingly, step up the flavor of low-calorie food and so can help win the battle of the bulge. With mustard, catsup and unsweetened pineapple juice you can make a wonderful sauce to use for barbecued baked chicken. Brown the chicken pieces in the oven first, drain off the accumulated fat, then spread each piece with sauce and continue to cook until chicken is crisp on the outside, tender within, about 45 to 50 minutes. A sauce made of mustard, currant jelly and beef stock is great over good-for-you pan-broiled calves liver; and mustard and chili sauce make for really great-tasting, stuffed, hard-cooked eggs.

These are only a few of the ways spices, seasoning and condiments can contribute to creative dieting, and you may be sure it is the only way you can change your eating pattern—not just a few useless weeks of dreary food but a lifetime eating style that will shed the pounds and, more importantly, keep them off forever with the bonus of beauty that is the result of supreme good health.

TWELVE TIPS THAT WILL HELP YOU STAY ON A DIET

1. Walk away from temptations. That's right. Resist the urge for a fattening snack or just that one piece of candy. Get out and walk even just five or six blocks. The fresh air will revive you and the change of scene will take your mind off food.

2. Make every meal a pleasurable event. Set the table attractively. Try to have fresh flowers. And leave your troubles somewhere else—nobody can enjoy food served with a litany of woes. Eat slowly and you will be satisfied with less food.

3. Instead of a bedtime snack take a marvelous warm bath. Make it special with fragrant bath salts, or, for dry, rough skin, add two cups of apple cider vinegar—or both. Invest in a loofah mat and scrub away rough, dry skin. Then just soak for a few minutes. Wrap yourself in a terry robe and get right into bed.

4. Take up some sort of sport. Swimming is one of the best. Every muscle gets a workout, but it's effortless as the water supports your body. Twenty minutes of swimming will burn up 100 calories.

5. Keep low-calorie snacks on hand—celery and carrot sticks, crisp apples, ripe tangerines. These are not only great appetite appeasers but good for you too.

6. Get involved. Plan some sort of activity for evenings and weekends. Every community has a public library. Take up a study of some segment of history if that appeals to you, or learn to play bridge or backgammon, or join a foreign-language class. In short, focus your attention on things other than food.

7. If you feel starved and it's hours before dinner, give yourself a great manicure with several coats of polish, allowing plenty of time for drying between each coat. You can't eat with wet polish on your nails.

8. If you have a problem skin with frequent "break-outs," invest in a trip to a dermatologist. Not only can he help clear up the condition, but he can reinforce your will to give up "junk" food, the prime cause of bad skin.

9. If, perchance, you have reached "that certain age" and wrinkles or a saggy, baggy face are making you unhappy, make an appointment now to get your face lifted. The plastic surgeon won't do it until you have lost any excess weight, so the determination can be a powerful incentive. Yes, it's expensive, but it's worth saving up for and you'll look so great you can economize by not having to buy more expensive, figure-hiding clothes. Even inexpensive skirts or pants are good on a slim figure.

10. Start taking a more active interest in your general appearance. New flattering makeup and a new hairstyle can help. Take pride in your hands and keep your nails well groomed. Give yourself a pedicure regularly. Your improved appearance by this consistent self-care will stiffen your diet willpower.

11. Your appetite can trick you into eating more food than you really want or need. The problem is that it takes about twenty minutes for the food you eat to start appeasing your desire for more. If you still feel hungry after a meal, don't go back for "seconds." Walk away from the table and start doing something else, clearing up the kitchen or whatever. In a half hour you won't feel hungry at all. Try it; it really works.

12. Keep portions small. There's no reason why you can't eat almost any good food you like if you cut down the amount. Don't heap your plate with food; take about half of what you normally eat. If you follow the suggestions above, you will quickly cut your appetite down to size.

10
Having It Your Way

Food is more than just nourishment. It's an emotional problem for most dieters. We all want more than just sufficient to appease our hunger, we want what we call "good-tasting" meals.

What tastes good to you, however, may not seem good to me—and there's the diet dilemma. Good-tasting food is a matter of opinion, based on emotions, because what most people relish is actually the food they are accustomed to eating. Taking away familiar food and substituting food that is different from customary fare makes most of us unhappy and dissatisfied.

That is why the recipes in this book relate to the meals most liked by the average American.

You can have it your way and still lose weight. It's just a matter of know-how.

When most of us plan a meal, whether simple or elaborate, first thoughts are about the meat course. We feel that dinner just isn't dinner if meat in some form is not included.

But can you lose weight on steak and potatoes? Yes, you can, with a little intelligent planning. Here's the proof positive, starting with America's most desired menu.

Broiled Flank Steak

Roasted Potatoes

Sliced Tomatoes Vinaigrette

Flank steak is a long, very lean piece of muscle from the belly of the steer. It usually weighs about 1½ lbs. from today's uniform animals. Its worth to dieters is its superb flavor but lack of fat. It is at its best prepared in the simplest of ways—brought to room temperature, then broiled quickly under a very hot flame, or better yet over a hot bed of glowing coals. For a steak that is nicely browned on the outside, rare and juicy within, broil close to heat for about 3 minutes on each side; more than that and this beef cut becomes dry, tough and stringy. Brush the meat before broiling with a little mild vegetable oil.

Before carving, sprinkle with a little top-quality dry sherry and generously with freshly ground black pepper. To carve, use a thin-bladed, very sharp knife and cut across the meat with the blade at a 20-degree angle to the surface. The slices will be about 3 inches in width and should be very thin. There will be sufficient to serve 3 to 4 slices to each of 3 to 4 hungry people (220 calories per 6-oz. serving).

Spoon over each serving some of the juice that has accumulated in the carving platter. It will taste divine. Salt, the only other seasoning necessary, may be added by each diner to suit his own taste.

This is one of the best steaks imaginable, and, though the price continues to rise as more and more people discover its qualities, it is still almost always less expensive than other beef steaks as well as lower in calories.

ROASTED POTATOES

Crisp on the outside, creamy smooth within. This is the way French-fried potatoes should taste—but so often they don't. They taste instead of the cooking oil used in their preparation and this flavor can be masked only by a heavy hand with the salt shaker and catsup bottle—both death to the dieter. But why go that route? Crisp-on-the-outside, creamy-inside potatoes are easier to come by, taste far better and are actually low calorie when they are oven-roasted.

Scrub large baking potatoes clean under cold running water. Blot dry and pierce in several places with the point of a small sharp knife. Place in a preheated 400° oven and bake for about 45 minutes or until they give a little when pressed gently and are almost—but not quite—soft.

Remove from oven; let stand for about 5 minutes, then cut in half lengthwise. Cut halves into 3 or 4 thick cubes. Place cubes on a baking sheet and broil, about 5 inches under the flame, until outsides of cubes are crisp and flecked with brown. Inside they will be soft and creamy. Sprinkle with a little salt 1 or 2 minutes before removing from the broiler (98 calories for each medium-size potato).

Twice as satisfying as fried potatoes, at half, or less, the calories, and you won't need catsup to hide the taste of the cooking oil.

TOMATOES VINAIGRETTE

How high in good flavor, low in calories can you get? Tomatoes sliced paper thin, marinated in just the right blend of oil, vinegar and seasoning might be your answer. Better for you than the usual mixed green salad, made palatable more often than not with blue cheese or other high-calorie dressing. Put thin slices of preferably vine-ripened tomatoes in a non-metal bowl. Sprinkle lightly, first with sugar—yes, sugar; it brings up the flavor—then salt and finally a mixture of three-quarters mild and fragrant safflower oil and one-quarter cider vinegar. Let stand in a cool place (but not in the refrigerator) for about an hour. Drain and sprinkle with minced parsley just before serving (medium-size tomato 40 calories). (Refrigerate to store if you must but, as tomatoes taste best just slightly cool, take them out of the "cold box" at least a half hour before serving.)

MORE ON AMERICA'S FAVORITE STEAK AND POTATOES

All steaks, despite most people's opinion, are not beef; a steak served often in Europe is veal. Really tender young veal is hard to come by in this country, but it can be had from a good butcher if ordered in advance and if you're willing to wait. You should be; it's worth it. It will undoubtedly be just as expensive as a fine fillet of beef, but it's superb eating, just as satisfying and contains about one-third less calories.

VEAL STEAKS PICATTA

Cooking is simplicity itself.
Have your butcher cut the steaks about ½-inch thick. Bring them to room temperature. Brush lightly with oil, then broil about 4 inches below broiler heat or over glowing coals for about 5 minutes per side. Serve on heated plates, accompanied by lemon wedges to squeeze over the meat, plus salt and black peppercorns to grind

from a peppermill directly onto the steak (4-oz. serving 250 calories).

For the total menu:

Veal Steaks Picatta

Stuffed Baked Potatoes

Zucchini Italian Style

You can prepare both potatoes and zucchini ahead and reheat them just before serving, making this one of the easiest of true diet-food meals.

STUFFED BAKED POTATOES

Scrub large baking potatoes clean under cold water. For crisp skins (shells that hold their shape for stuffing), rub each potato lightly with vegetable oil. Pierce them lightly in several places with the tip of a small knife. Bake in a 350° oven until done (97 calories per medium-size before stuffing potato). To test, wrap your hand in a clean kitchen towel and press the potato gently; it should "give" easily under light pressure.

Remove from the oven, cut in half lengthwise and scoop out centers into a mixing bowl. Set skin shells aside. For each potato add one heaping tablespoon of cottage cheese and about 3 tbs. of skim milk. (Have the cheese and skim milk at room temperature or they will chill the potato.) Mash, then beat the mixture until it is completely free of lumps. Add additional milk if needed. Ideally it should be neither wet nor dry and should hold its shape lightly when scooped up in a spoon. Add, for each potato about 1 tbs. grated Swiss cheese (lower in calories than grated Parmesan but equally flavorful) and season to taste with salt.

Fill the potato shells with the mixture and either set aside or store in the refrigerator until ready for final baking. Or freeze until firm, wrap in airtight freezer wrap and store in freezer until needed. For final baking place in preheated 400° oven until thoroughly heated. Each stuffed one-half baked potato about 100 calories.

ZUCCHINI ITALIAN STYLE

Chop two unpeeled ripe and juicy tomatoes (for each 4 servings) in a heavy skillet, letting the released juices fall into the skillet. Cook over low heat, chopping the tomatoes still further as they cook until they are reduced to a chunky but liquidy sauce.

Wash, trim and thinly slice 1 medium-size zucchini for each serving and add it to the tomato sauce. Season with salt, a bit of hot-pepper sauce and a sprinkling of black pepper. Cover and simmer until zucchini is tender. Add a little water if mixture becomes too dry. Thicken the sauce with a few soft bread crumbs made from fresh Italian-style bread and a teaspoon or so of grated Parmesan cheese.

This is a hearty and filling vegetable dish, yet in spite of bread crumbs and cheese it can be rated as calorie low (59 calories per serving).

But why limit your steak to meat only? Many fish make great "steak" dinners. One of the best is salmon. It's a hearty fish, and makes a filling meal when teamed with tiny steamed new potatoes and spinach with water chestnuts. It's a menu even the most dedicated beef eaters will want to repeat.

*Salmon Steaks
with Lemon Sauce*

Steamed New Potatoes

*Spinach with
Water Chestnuts and Soy Sauce*

SALMON STEAKS

Pour into a deep 10-inch skillet about 2 cups water, ½ cup dry white wine, 1 tbs. lemon juice and 1 tbs. crab boil (a blend of spices you'll find on your grocers' spice shelf—if not available, substitute a bay leaf and a pinch of thyme). Bring mixture to a boil, then lower heat and simmer for about 30 minutes. Add 2 to 4 one-inch-thick salmon steaks (one for each serving). Cover and poach for about 15 minutes or until they flake easily when touched with a fork. Remove with a spatula, drain and place on serving plates.

While salmon cooks prepare the sauce by combining for each 2 servings 3 tbs. olive oil, 2 tbs. lemon juice and 1 tbs. water. Blend and add salt to taste. Pour into a small non-metal saucepan. Beat, heat and pour over salmon steaks when they are ready to come to the table. (Salmon 179 calories per serving. Sauce 192 calories per serving.)

STEAMED NEW POTATOES

You'll want the smallest new potatoes you can find and they should be, as nearly as possible, all the same size. Scrub them clean under cold water and place them, unpeeled, in a single layer in a 10-inch skillet. Add a bit of butter (1 tbs. for 8 to 12 very tiny potatoes) and pour in water to the depth of about 1 inch. Cover and steam the potatoes in the liquid over medium heat until tender. If they are really small, about 15 minutes will do the job nicely. Shake the pan often so that the potatoes roll around in the liquid, but uncover as little as you dare so that the steam doesn't escape. Add more water if all boils away, but hopefully you won't have to do so; the pan should be almost dry when the potatoes are cooked. Sprinkle lightly with salt. (About 140 calories per serving of each 3 to 4 potatoes.)

SPINACH WITH WATER CHESTNUTS

Wash 2 lbs. tender young spinach. Remove tough stems and wash again under cold running water. Place in a medium saucepan with only the water that clings to the leaves. Cover the pan and place over medium heat. When the cover is hot, reduce the heat to low and cook for five minutes. Uncover, drain and stir in 6 to 8 coarsely chopped, well-drained water chestnuts and 1 tsp. fresh lemon juice. Season with about 1 tsp. soy sauce, and stir-fry for about 1 minute to heat thoroughly just before serving (about 100 calories per serving).

11
Creative Dieting

LITTLE LUXURIES TO KEEP YOU HAPPILY ON A DIET

Here is a list of little "extras" that make a low-calorie diet fun, not painful. Yes, they are expensive, but so is the doctor, and the extras are much pleasanter. Also, the right diet that is nutritionally sound will eliminate your need to buy painkillers, laxatives, mouthwash, antacid preparations or deodorants. A healthy non-toxic system doesn't need any of them and you will find it much more satisfying to spend the money saved on any or all of the following items.

Caviar
The red variety is delicious and not fabulously high priced.
Granular 1 oz 74 calories. Pressed 1 oz 89.

Good Cheese
Don't forget a really great Swiss cheese. It's low-calorie and makes a great snack or, with a piece of ripe fruit, a perfect lunch (about 100 calories per ounce).

Imported Crackers
English water biscuits (61 calories each), wheat wafers (22 calories each), et cetera.

Luxurious Cookies
Try crisp, delicate French gaufrettes. These little V-shaped morsels are so good that one turns an afternoon cup of tea into a special treat. (Close the tin firmly after one.)

Fresh Oysters
Begin dinner with six oysters on the half shell accompanied by a really hot horseradish-spiked cocktail sauce and a dash of fresh lemon. Or broil them, in the shell if possible, for an elegant dinner of soup, then broiled oysters, followed by fresh fruit and cheese for dessert. Despite their luxurious taste, oysters are almost zero calories, yet very filling.

Super Fruit
There are any number of companies that will ship spectacular fruit to you each month. Big juicy grapefruit (about 100 calories), oranges (about 75 calories) and tangerines (about 39 calories) from Texas. Huge ripe pears (100 calories each), and beautiful seedless grapes (½ cup, 48 calories) from Oregon. Yes, they are expensive but worth it.

Special Honey
Experiment. There are all sorts of extra-delicious, raw honeys from France and Switzerland that are especially delicious and will make you forget you ever wanted sugar. Honey is much sweeter than sugar so "less" is happily "more " (64 calories in 1 tablespoon).

Wild Rice
Yes, it is fabulously expensive, but a little goes a long way and, like all whole natural grain, it is rich in vitamins and minerals. Try it with Ris de Veau Marchand du Vin or with French Roast Chicken. It's so luxurious it's almost sinful (½ cup, 73 calories).

Big English Cocktail Onions
These are so good few people can stop eating them. Since they are calorie free, go ahead. Enjoy—enjoy!

Really Good Pepper
Black Java pepper is expensive, but the flavor bonus is fantastic and per dish it's only a few pennies extra (no calories).

Smoked Salmon
Lovely for an epicurean first course or as an entrée for a summer lunch. Serve with cucumber slices and plenty of capers (2 ozs., 100 calories).

Pickled Herring
Buy one of the better brands. Serve it for lunch on crisp leaves of Boston lettuce. Low calorie and rich in vitamins, iron and calcium (2 ozs., 125 calories).

Fine Tea
A lovely little luxury that makes an afternoon cup of tea an event. It's fun to experiment with different teas. Smoky Hu Kwah tea in its black tin box is one of my favorites. Expensive but worth every penny. Order from Bloomingdale's Delicacy Dept., Lexington Avenue at 59th St., New York, N.Y. 10021 if not locally available (1 cup, 1 calorie).

Fine Cognac
Plus a bottle of kirsch and Grand Marnier. Quite a little investment, but a few drops transform fruit desserts into "specials" and a drop or two in a small cup of black coffee makes a luxurious ending to dinner. You won't miss the sugar at all (1 tbs., 40 calories).

Add your own special favorites. The big thing is to stay with a diet and a few "extras" are a big help. Try the idea and see if it doesn't work. Of course it does.

Crème Fraiche
The cultured heavy cream the French have long used in cooking or served with fresh fruit, particularly raspberries or strawberries, is now available in this country. Hopefully by the time you read this it will be readily purchased in your area. However, if it's not available in your locality, it's easily made at home and, while it is loaded with calories, it's actually a calorie cutter when used for cooking in the French manner. One tablespoon will thicken the same amount of sauce as 3 tablespoons of butter mixed with three tablespoons of flour. For a change of pace, it may be substituted for yogurt in any of the sauce recipes included in this book. For a delicate and delectable green-bean casserole that's good enough to serve as a luncheon main course try the recipe on page 194.
To make your own Crème Fraiche simply combine 1 cup of heavy cream and 2 tablespoons of buttermilk in a jar with a tight-fitting screw-top lid. Shake well to mix thoroughly and place in a warm place, such as a sunny window. It will thicken to the consistency of sour cream in 24 to 36 hours, depending on temperature. Once thickened, refrigerate until needed. Keeps well for at least two weeks (56 calories per tbs.).

Menus and Recipes

12
The Cocktail Hour

Of course you want to cut out hard liquor both for health and weight loss, but if you are used to a pre-dinner drink accompanied by some sort of tasty hors d'oeuvres, it's hard to break the habit. It's a social hour that is a pleasant, relaxing time of the day and can be sorely missed. Well, take heart. There are low-calorie drinks and accompanying snacks that can replace hard liquor and that forbidden fattening "something to go with." Try the recipe (on page 106) for a Bloodless Mary, or have a glass of sparkly Perrier water with a slice of lime. Then there are wine coolers, low in alcohol and wonderfully refreshing on a warm evening. Even a glass of dry sherry, preferably served on the rocks, is not too high in either alcohol or calories to be forbidden. And for a festive occasion a glass of champagne is still far less fattening than a martini or Scotch on the rocks.

There are any number of low-calorie hors d'oeuvres to add zest to the cocktail hour without adding pounds on you. Try the recipe for Yogurt Vegetable Dip (page 112), or (page 113) for crisp baked potato skins. (What to do with the inside is included.)

Still another energy-packed, good-for-you idea is Guacamole (page 111), made with ripe avocados and spread on paper-thin whole-wheat wafers. As mentioned

previously raw turnip slices are great for spreading with
cheddar cheese, and celery stalks, stuffed with creamed
cottage cheese mixed with appropriate seasoning can be
a delicious and satisfying snack.

Actually, when you get right down to it, these are far
more satisfying than potato chips, nuts or other high-
calorie cocktail fare. As with all food, it is important that
everything you eat should contribute not to excess
weight but to vitality and good nutrition and, while this
may sound dull, the high-energy vitality foods actually
taste far better than processed junk.

Elizabeth Arden, one of the pioneers in beautiful
weight loss, worked out the menus and recipes for her
famed Maine Chance beauty resort with Gayelord Hauser
way back in the thirties and his principle still holds true
today. The potato-skin recipe (potato crisps, p. 113) was
his original idea and he instituted the glass of fruit or
vegetable juice in place of the pre-dinner cocktail.
Today, in his eighties, Hauser has the face and body of a
well-trimmed fifty-five, living proof of what a lifetime of
good and good-for-you food can do to achieve and
maintain a beautiful you all the years of your life.

BLOODLESS MARY

Juice of ½ lime
1 cup tomato juice
Dash of
Worcestershire
Dash of Tabasco
Small stalk of celery

For each serving combine all the ingredients except
celery and pour over ice cubes. Garnish with celery stalk
(61 calories per serving).

WINE COOLER

½ cup dry red wine
Juice of ½ orange

Combine in a tall glass, add ice cubes. Fill with sparkling water—and enjoy (115 calories).

APERITIFS AND SODA

Use half your favorite aperitif, half soda, over lots of ice. Add a twist of lemon peel if you like.

The following aperitifs are good choices: Dubonnet, Lillet, Byrrh, sweet or dry vermouth (about 65 to 75 calories per 8-oz. glass).

AMERICANO

2 jiggers sweet   1 jigger Campari
  vermouth

Combine in a tall glass over ice cubes. Fill with soda. Add a twist of lemon peel (128 calories).

Vermouth, particularly the dry vermouth, makes an admirable substitute for higher-calorie drinks. Just pour it over the rocks and add a twist of lemon peel.

Tonic water too, poured over ice and garnished with a slice of lime, is wonderful on a warm evening.

SEAFOOD APPETIZERS

You can cut your appetite for dinner considerably if you take time out for a low-calorie drink and a substantial but non-fattening appetizer. The best one of all is a cold shrimp-and-crab-claw platter and it's festive enough to make a great choice for a party.

Or just a bowl of cold boiled shrimp ready for dunking into a spicy cocktail or Rémoulade sauce. Yes, shrimp and crab claws are expensive, but it's easy enough to follow this kind of appetizer with a supper of delicious but inexpensive soup and a dessert of fresh fruit. It makes for a wonderfully well-balanced and great-tasting meal.

RÉMOULADE SAUCE

½ cup mayonnaise
½ cup chili sauce
1 tbs. lemon juice
2 tbs. finely chopped sweet pickles

1 tbs. capers
1 tsp. grated onion

Combine all ingredients and blend well. Refrigerate until served (about 140 calories per tbs., sufficient for 1 serving).

CAPONATA

1 medium eggplant (about 1 lb.)
Salt
1 tbs. olive oil
2 tbs. safflower oil
1 large mild onion, peeled and chopped

4 to 6 celery stalks, finely chopped
1 small carrot, scraped and finely chopped
1 or 2 cloves garlic, peeled and finely minced

1 one-lb. can Italian plum tomatoes, drained and chopped (save juice for soups and sauces)

1 tbs. tomato paste

4 oil-cured black olives, pitted and slivered

3 tbs. red wine vinegar

1 3- to 3½-oz. tin anchovy fillets, drained and minced Freshly ground black pepper

1 tsp. sugar

¼ to ½ cup finely minced parsley

Peel eggplant and cut into small cubes. Sprinkle generously with salt and spread on paper toweling. Cover with more paper toweling and weigh down with heavy plate. Let stand for 30 minutes. Rinse off salt; pat cubes dry.

Heat oils together in heavy 10-inch skillet and add onion, celery, carrot and garlic. Cook over low heat, stirring frequently, until vegetables are tender. Add the remaining ingredients, except the parsley. Stir to blend and bring to a boil. Lower heat and simmer gently until eggplant cubes are tender but still holding their shape. Spoon into serving dish and cool to room temperature. Stir in parsley just before serving.

6 to 8 servings as part of an antipasto platter. As an appetizer 8 to 10 servings.

Can be made ahead, if you wish. Refrigerate covered, but remove from refrigerator about 30 minutes before serving as Caponata tastes best just slightly chilled or at room temperature. 80 to 104 calories per serving depending on size of serving.

Asparagus Maltaise

Perfect as a first course for dinner or as a luncheon entrée.

STEAMED ASPARAGUS

6 to 8 asparagus stalks   Pimiento strips
   per serving
   Sauce Maltaise (see
   below)

Rinse asparagus under cold water. Cut off the tough, woody ends. Then, with a vegetable peeler, peel from the tip down, rolling the stalks around as you work. Rinse again. The peeling, which should actually be only a light scraping, gets rid of all sand and makes the whole stalk tender and eatable.

Arrange the asparagus stalks on a rack (I use a cake rack in a 12-inch skillet) and spread out in a single layer so that they will cook evenly. (Rectangular vegetable steamers with racks are available and are perfect for steaming all vegetables.)

Fill the bottom of your skillet or steamer with about 1½ inches of water. Add asparagus. Cover, place over medium-high heat and steam until tender. Time depends on the thickness of the asparagus stalks, but they are done when they can be pierced easily with the tip of a small knife. This usually takes only 5 to 8 minutes. Don't overcook or they will be limp and flavorless. Add a little more boiling water if necessary.

Rinse immediately with cold water and stop cooking process. Asparagus need not be hot as an accompanying vegetable, but is actually best when served at room temperature.

Arrange on small (salad-size) plates, top each serving with a bit (about 2 tbs.) of cold Sauce Maltaise and garnish with a thin strip of pimiento (about 155 calories per serving).

SAUCE MALTAISE

1 tbs. mayonnaise (see recipe page 210-11)	1 tbs. freshly squeezed (strained) orange juice
1 tsp. yogurt	Pinch of grated orange or lemon rind

Blend well and spoon over asparagus just before serving (126 calories per serving).

GUACAMOLE

1 large ripe avocado	1 tsp. cumin seeds
1 tbs. lemon juice	(optional)
1 tbs. grated onion	2 or 3 dashes Tabasco

Peel and mash avocado until light and smooth. Blend in lemon juice and seasonings. If prepared ahead, place the avocado pit in mixture to prevent darkening.

Cover and refrigerate until ready to serve.

Serves 4 to 6 as a dip (82 calories per serving for 4; 55 calories per serving for 6).

CURRY GARLIC DIP FOR CRUDITIES

¾ cup mayonnaise	Salt
¾ cup yogurt	Freshly ground black pepper
1 or 2 cloves garlic, peeled and put through a press	1 to 2 tbs. fresh lemon juice
1 to 2 tsps. good quality imported curry powder	1 to 3 tbs. light rum

Combine mayonnaise, yogurt, garlic and curry powder. Blend well. Flavor with salt, pepper, lemon juice and rum. Let stand about 1 hour at room temperature to develop flavor, then refrigerate until time to serve. Correct seasoning as needed.

Makes about 1½ cups, about 50 calories per serving.

NOTE: Crudities tray might include peeled thinly sliced raw turnip and unpeeled zucchini (keep in icy lemon bath, juice of ½ lemon and 2 cups icy-cold water to preserve color until ready to serve), cauliflower flowerettes, carrot sticks, celery stalks and cherry tomatoes.

YOGURT VEGETABLE DIP

1 container plain yogurt
2 tbs. finely minced celery
2 tbs. finely minced green pepper

1 tbs. grated onion
Dash Tabasco

Blend all ingredients and chill before serving.
6 servings (about 25 calories per serving).

STUFFED CELERY

½ cup cottage cheese
¼ cup grated sharp cheddar cheese
1 tbs. chopped pimento

¼ cup milk
6 to 8 stalks green celery

Combine ingredients except celery and place in electric blender. Blend until smooth. Fill celery stalks with mixture and chill until ready to serve (about 36 calories each).

POTATO CRISPS
WITH A CREAMED-POTATO BONUS

3 large baking potatoes   Salt
(blemish-free skins
please)

Preheat oven to 375°.

Wash potatoes thoroughly, pierce skins in several spots with the point of a small knife. Bake in preheated oven until soft. About 1 hour. Slice potatoes in half lengthwise, scoop out inside into a bowl and set aside.

Cut skins into quarters, sprinkle lightly with salt and return to oven for about 5 minutes or until crisp and dry. Fabulously good with any sort of drink, low calorie and rich with vitamins (about 5 calories per serving, allowing 2 Crisps for each serving).

CREAMED POTATOES

While potato skins are baking prepare creamed potatoes.

Preheat oven to 375°.

Potatoes leftover from   2 tbs. Parmesan cheese
potato crisps   Salt
¼ cup milk   Freshly ground black
½ cup yogurt   pepper

Mash potatoes thoroughly with milk, yogurt and Parmesan cheese until smooth and light. Season to taste with salt and pepper, spoon into lightly buttered casserole and bake in preheated oven for about 20 minutes or until very hot.* Serve at once.

4 servings (115 calories per serving).

ESCABECHE

1 large mild onion, peeled and sliced
2 cloves garlic, peeled and cut in half lengthwise
1 bay leaf
1 cup red wine vinegar
½ tsp. salt
6 to 8 peppercorns
1 cup olive oil

2 lbs. cod or halibut fillets
Boston lettuce leaves
1 avocado, cut in half, seed removed, each half peeled, cut into thin slices and sprinkled with lemon juice
Pimiento strips

To prepare marinade: Combine onion, garlic, bay leaf and vinegar in a medium saucepan. Bring to a boil, lower heat and simmer until onion is soft. Add salt and peppercorns. Cool, then add ¾ cup of the oil. Set aside.

Cut each fillet into 2-inch strips. Heat the remaining oil in a 10- to 12-inch skillet. In it cook the fish strips in a single layer, for about 1 minute on each side (only until firm and white). Don't overcook. If all strips do not fit into the pan in one layer, cook in stages, adding more oil if needed. Transfer the strips as cooked to a long, shallow glass or ceramic dish. When all are done, pour the marinade over them. Cover and refrigerate for 12 to 24 hours.

Drain and arrange marinated fish strips on leaves of

* Note: May be prepared ahead and stored, covered, in the refrigerator until ready to bake.

crisp lettuce. Garnish with slices of acvocado and pimiento strips.

Serves 6 to 8 as a first-course appetizer or the drained fish strips may be served as part of an antipasto platter (80 to 100 calories per serving).

MARINATED MUSHROOMS

1 lb. fresh mushrooms
1 large onion, peeled and chopped
2 cloves garlic, peeled and minced
2 bay leaves
Freshly ground pepper
Salt

1 cup dry white wine
½ cup tarragon vinegar
¼ cup safflower oil or corn oil
1 tbs. lemon juice
¼ cup minced parsley

Wipe mushrooms clean with a damp cloth. Trim off stems. Combine with remaining ingredients in an enamelized or glass saucepan. Bring to a boil, then reduce heat and simmer for about 10 minutes, stirring frequently. Cool in the cooking liquid, then refrigerate for several hours (or, if you wish, for several days).

To serve, drain. Spear each mushroom with a food pick and serve as an appetizer or add to an antipasto platter (about 20 calories per serving of 6 to 8 mushrooms).

13
Soup, Beautiful Soup

Soup can be the weight loser's best ally, filling, nourishing and calorie low. When made with imagination, using good basic stock and just a little care, it is also the gourmet's favorite for a luncheon or supper. As for work, there's very little of it with stock on hand. A rich-tasting super soup can be made in short order with chicken or beef stock. What's more to the point, it's a dieter's dream, low in calories and high in appetite satisfaction. But don't spoil the game with doughy, salty crackers. Substitute thin little crisp Italian breadsticks or whole-grain rice or wheat wafers. Both are generally available, lower calorie than crackers, and a lot better with soup anyway.

CLASSIC ONION SOUP

One of the all-time-great soups, pure heaven on a cold winter night, a sturdy onion soup is easy to make and a satisfying yet still calorie-low choice for supper. Add a fresh spinach salad and, for dessert, a serving of pears poached in red wine.

2 tbs. butter	4 slices toasted French
4 onions, peeled and thinly sliced	bread
2 tsps. flour	2 ozs. grated Swiss cheese
5 cups clear fat-free chicken stock, heated	

Melt the butter in a large saucepan over very low heat. Add onion slices, cover, and cook slowly over very low heat until they are soft and translucent, but not brown. Add the flour, stir to blend and cook, still over low heat, for 2 or 3 minutes. Add chicken stock, stir to blend and simmer for about 30 minutes. Preheat oven to 375°. Pour soup into ovenproof bowls, top with toasted French bread, sprinkle with grated cheese and place in oven for a few minutes until cheese melts. Serve at once.

4 servings (about 250 calories per serving).

BORSCH

This is beautiful soup, its deep red color contrasting with a snowy spoonful of yogurt and enlivened (if the budget permits) with a sprinkling of red or black caviar. Simple and quick to make, it is delicious served hot or icy cold and an excellent beginning for a dinner party winter or summer. Low-calorie fare with a flair.

2 cups of freshly cooked
  beets, peeled and
  chopped (Canned
  beets may be
  substituted if desired.)
4 cups clear, fat-free
  chicken stock
1 tbs. butter
1 small onion, finely
  minced

2 stalks celery, finely
  minced
1 tbs. lemon juice
  Salt
  Freshly ground black
  pepper
  Yogurt
  Red or black caviar
  (optional)

Place the beets and ½ cup of the chicken stock in an electric blender and blend to a purée at high speed.

Melt the butter in a large saucepan and sauté the onion and celery over very low heat until limp but not brown. Add the puréed beets and remaining chicken stock. Simmer for 25 to 30 minutes. Stir in lemon juice, season with salt and pepper. Serve very hot or chill until very cold. In either case garnish with a spoonful of yogurt and, if possible, a sprinkling of caviar.

4 to 6 servings about 185 calories per serving for 4; about 120 calories per serving for 6.

SPINACH SOUP

This is a delicate fresh-tasting soup that makes for a perfect lunch. A fresh ripe pear and a wedge of Camembert cheese makes a perfect dessert and who could ask for more, dieter or non-dieter.

1 lb. fresh spinach (You can substitute 1 package of frozen spinach, but fresh does taste better.)	1 clove garlic, peeled and finely minced
5½ cups chicken stock	Salt
2 tbs. butter	Freshly ground black pepper
½ cup minced green onions	Grated nutmeg (optional)

Wash the spinach thoroughly to rid it of any sand. Place in a medium saucepan with ½ cup of the chicken stock. Cover and cook briefly, only until tender (about 5 to 10 minutes). Place spinach and cooking liquid in an electric blender and blend to a purée.

Melt butter in a large saucepan over low heat and sauté onion and garlic until limp but not brown. Add spinach purée and remaining chicken stock. Bring to a boil, then reduce heat and simmer, uncovered, for 15 to 20 minutes. Season to taste and serve hot.

6 servings (about 95 calories per serving).

The beauty of this soup is its fresh taste. It does not do well as a leftover. If you want a smaller quantity, the recipe may easily be cut in half.

GAZPACHO

Now, this really is a soup for the gourmet. The fact that it is low calorie—and very good for you with its plentiful use of raw vegetables—is a plus, but the real idea is that it makes for a super-perfect summer-day lunch or Sunday-night supper. It is so calorie low that you might splurge on a fairly rich dessert. A small cup of black coffee as a finale.

1 cup dry white wine	1 clove garlic, peeled
½ tsp. black peppercorns	and minced
2 tsps. chopped fresh	
basil (1 tsp. crushed	
dried basil may be	
substituted if the fresh	
is not available)	

Combine all the above ingredients in a small non-metal saucepan and simmer until reduced to about ½ cup. Set aside to cool.

4 cups strong fat-free	¼ cup chopped celery
stock	Salt
1 tsp. lemon juice	Freshly ground black
4 ripe tomatoes, peeled,	pepper
seeded and finely	Garlic-flavored
chopped	croutons (optional)
1 cucumber, peeled and	4 to 6 per serving
finely chopped	

Bring stock to a boil, then transfer to a non-metal bowl. Strain the wine mixture and add to the stock. Allow to cool, then add lemon juice and vegetables. Chill until very cold. Season to taste with salt and pepper. Serve in chilled soup cups. Garnish if desired with a few garlic croutons.

Serves 6 (about 60 calories per serving).

NOTE: In Spain a little olive oil is added to the chilled soup, but in my opinion it does not add to the flavor, only to the calorie count.

SOUP OF THE DAY: VEGETABLE MÉLANGE

Make enough for a crowd or for one serving. Use any or all of the following in any quantity desired.

Mushroom stems, trimmed and chopped
Celery, sliced, including the green leaves
Green onions, trimmed and chopped
Yellow squash or zucchini, trimmed, unpeeled, but chopped or sliced
Carrots, scraped and sliced or chopped
Potato, peeled and chopped
Half and half water and clear fat-free chicken or beef stock (homemade stock or, if you must, canned)
Salt
Spinach leaves, chopped parsley, and snow pea pods (optional)

Use about 1 cup total vegetables for each two cups of liquid. Place all vegetables (except spinach leaves and snow pea pods) and liquid in a large heavy pot and simmer until vegetables are tender. Season with salt to taste. (Can, of course, be made ahead and reheated.)

Now add, if you like, a handful of chopped fresh spinach leaves, some chopped parsley and a few pea pods and simmer for a few additional minutes.

With crusty bread and a small glass of wine, this makes a great and hearty but low-calorie meal. (Calories depend on vegetables used, but, no matter how generous, a goodly portion loaded with vegetables can't exceed 100 calories.)

A QUICK-TO-THE TABLE
COUNTRY FISH CHOWDER

2 tbs. butter
1 large onion, peeled
  and coarsely chopped
3 large potatoes
  (California white
  potatoes are best),
  peeled and coarsely
  chopped
4 cups water

2 cups (bottled) clam
  juice
2 lbs. fillet of flounder,
  cut into 2-inch-wide
  pieces
  Freshly ground black
  pepper
  Salt
¼ cup minced parsley

Melt the butter in a soup pot over low heat. Add the onion and potatoes and cook, stirring often, for about 5 minutes. Add the water and clam juice and simmer until potatoes are tender.

Add the flounder. Cover and cook for about 5 minutes or until fish flakes easily when touched with a fork. Sprinkle generously with pepper to taste and add salt only as needed (clam juice is salty). Stir in parsley and serve very hot in shallow soup bowls.

Serves 4 (about 300 calories per serving).

TWENTY-MINUTE HEARTY BEEF AND VEGETABLE SOUP

1 tbs. olive oil
1 medium-size onion,
  peeled and chopped
1 small green pepper,
  seeded, all white fiber
  removed and pepper
  chopped
2 stalks celery with
  leaves, chopped
1 large ripe tomato,
  peeled, seeded and
  chopped

4 cups water
¾ lb. top round of beef,
  all fat removed, and
  meat ground twice
1 cup cold (leftover)
  cooked rice
  Pinch dried oregano
  Salt
  Red-hot pepper flakes

Heat the olive oil in a soup pot. Add onion, green pepper and celery. Cook, stirring, over low heat until vegetables are tender. Add tomato and cook, chopping the pieces still further with the tip of a spatula until they are quite soft. Add water and bring to a boil. Add beef and rice and simmer soup for about 10 minutes. Season with oregano and salt. Add hot-pepper flakes to taste.

Serves 4 to 6 (4 servings, about 235 calories per serving; 6 servings, about 155 calories per serving).

POTATO-CHIVE SOUP

4 to 6 medium-size
  potatoes, peeled and
  chopped
5 cups chicken stock
¼ cup minced fresh
  chives
  Pinch dried rosemary
  (optional)

2 egg yolks
1 tbs. Half & Half
¼ cup dry sherry
  Salt

Cook potatoes in stock over low heat until they are very soft.

Purée in container of electric blender (you will have to do this in 3 batches). Transfer as puréed to a second pot and add chives. Bring to simmering and cook, stirring, for 2 to 3 minutes, until very hot.

Combine egg yolks, cream and sherry and beat until well blended. Add about ½ cup of the hot potato soup, beating briskly as added.

Remove soup from heat and stir egg-yolk mixture rapidly into the soup. Salt to taste. Ladle into heated soup bowls and serve at once.

Serves 4 to 6 (about 225 calories per serving for 4; about 150 calories per serving for 6).

CREAM OF TOMATO SOUP

This is the best tomato soup I have ever had. Hearty and flavorful, it is extremely low calorie and when served with Italian breadsticks, followed by cheese and fruit for dessert, makes a great luncheon or supper.

6 large ripe tomatoes	1 tsp. freshly ground
1 small onion, peeled	black pepper
and chopped	1 tsp. basil, fresh if
6 cups fat-free chicken	possible
stock	2 tbs. Crème Fraiche
1 tsp. salt	(see recipe page 102)

Dip tomatoes into boiling water for a moment, then slip off the skins with the point of a sharp knife. Cut into chunks and place tomatoes and onions in a blender. Blend to a purée at high speed. Combine with stock and seasonings in a medium saucepan. Bring to a boil, lower heat and simmer for about 20 minutes. Remove from heat, stir in Crème Fraiche and blend well. Serve very hot.

6 servings (about 95 calories per serving).

JELLIED BORSCH

1 envelope unflavored gelatin
½ cup cold water
2 cups fat-free beef stock or broth
2 cooked fresh beets, peeled and chopped, well drained (see below)

1 tbs. fresh lemon juice
1 tbs. prepared horseradish
Sour cream, or yogurt (optional)

Soften gelatin in cold water. Heat stock to boiling. Add softened gelatin and stir over low heat until dissolved.

Combine remaining ingredients in a bowl. Pour in stock mixture and stir until blended. Chill until thickened.

Serve in chilled cups, topped, if you like, with a bit of sour cream or plain yogurt.

6 servings. (With yogurt 25 to 30 calories per serving. With sour cream about 250 calories per serving.)

NOTE: To prepare beets retaining all nutrients: Wash beets and bake on a rack in a 350° oven until they can be easily pierced through center with a small kitchen knife. Scrub off peel, holding each beet under cold water.

14
Stock and Sauces

BEEF STOCK

You can omit the celery and mushroom stems from the following recipe if you must, but they do add immeasurably to the stock's flavor. The next time you buy mushrooms, reserve the stems. Pack them in a tightly closed plastic bag and freeze until you are ready to make your stock.

Now for several tips on stock-making. There's nothing to it really. It must simmer for hours, but you don't have to simmer along with it. It should cook, uncovered, over very, very low heat. Use an asbestos pad over the flame if necessary. If the stock boils, it will not be clear. Stock is done when it takes on a shiny, almost syrupy, look. Cool uncovered. If it is covered while cooling, it will take on a sour taste.

3	lbs. shank of beef (bone in)	½	green pepper
1	veal knuckle bone (if not available, substitute 1 lb. of oxtails)	½	cup mushroom stems
		4	cloves garlic, peeled
		1	small bunch parsley
		1	or 2 stalks of celery, leaves included
1	pig's foot (optional but desirable)	2	cups dry red wine
2	medium onions, peeled and cut in half	1	tsp. salt
			Water as required
3	to 4 carrots, scraped and washed		

Preheat oven to 375.°

Place beef shanks and bones in a large heavy kettle, (enamelized cast iron is best). Place in preheated oven for 20 to 30 minutes or until meat and bones are brown. Place kettle on top of stove. Add remaining ingredients and enough water to come to about 1 inch from rim of kettle. Bring to a boil, then lower heat so that stock barely simmers. Cook, uncovered, for 6 to 8 hours, adding more water to keep pot about one-half full.

When stock is done, cool, uncovered, then strain into a large bowl, discarding bones and vegetables but reserving meat for cold beef with horseradish sauce (see recipe page 157). Refrigerate stock until fat has risen and congealed on the surface. Remove and discard fat.

If properly made, stock will have jellied somewhat and can be ladled into pint-size Mason jars for easy storing or, if not to be used within two or three days, it should be frozen to use whenever needed. To remove frozen stock place the container in a pan of cold water until sufficiently thawed.

About 30 calories per cup.

QUICK BEEF STOCK
(using canned beef broth)

There really is no substitute for a homemade, well-made stock, but if there is none on hand, you need not resort to fattening ingredients such as butter, cream or milk. Instead use canned broth. Some of the better brands (though not as good or good for you as homemade) are sufficiently good to use directly from the can, but they can be considerably improved in flavor with a bit of preliminary treatment. Simmering canned broth with a bit of wine and a few odds and ends of vegetables will almost completely remove the "canned" taste.

Here are two "loose" recipes. You can, of course, change them a bit to accommodate "what's on hand" in your kitchen.

2 eight-oz. cans condensed beef broth	2 or 3 sprigs parsley
½ cup Madeira	2 or 3 stalks celery with leaves
2 cups water	Several mushroom stems, trimmed and chopped
1 small onion, peeled and sliced	
1 clove garlic, peeled and minced	1 bay leaf

Combine all ingredients in a heavy medium saucepan. Bring to a full boil, then lower heat and simmer for about 30 minutes.

Strain before using.

Makes about 3 cups stock (about 30 calories per cup).

GRAVY

You can make a low-calorie but thick, rich meat gravy for steak, chops or leftover slices of roast meat without using that seemingly indispensable rendered meat fat or other fat, blended with flour and thinned with high-calorie milk or tasteless water.

Start with your own flavorful homemade beef stock. (If you must, use canned clear beef stock, but the gravy just won't be as good.) For each cup of stock add 2 tbs. flour and whirl until smooth in an electric blender, or shake in a jar with a tight-fitting lid until smooth.

If you have it, add 2 or 3 tbs. of what the French call *le jus*, saved from the roast. This is the rich meat essence that drips, as a roast cooks, into the bottom of the roasting pan along with the fat from the meat. To remove the fat: After the roast has been transferred to a serving platter, pour the liquid contents of the roasting pan into a refrigerator dish and chill until all fat has risen to the surface and congealed. What is left underneath are the deep-protein-rich drippings—*le jus*—and no bottled steak sauce, no other seasoning, can give such a deep-down-good flavor to your gravy.

Pour well-blended stock, flour and *le jus* into an 8- to 10-inch heavy skillet and stir over low heat until thickened. Add salt and pepper to taste,.

A superb sauce for steak, leftover roast beef or pot roast requires only two ingredients: homemade beef stock and a bit of dry Madeira, about 2 tablespoons of Madeira for each cup of stock. Remove and discard all fat from stock. Add Madeira and simmer over low heat until reduced to a naturally thick glaze. Season with salt and pepper and that's all there is to it but it tastes great. About 80 calories per cup. For sliced, boiled tongue add a teaspoon of currant jelly and cook, stirring, until smooth. With jelly, about 10 additional calories per cup.

CHICKEN STOCK

Made in almost the same manner as beef stock, chicken stock is a marvelous addition to your culinary repertoire. Used as the cooking liquid for any stir-fried dish of chicken or seafood, or as a low-calorie base for creamed food or curry, it adds not just powerful nutrition but infinite flavor. Quick-cooking recipes take on an "hours-of-preparation" taste when you cook with stock.

1	three to three-and-a-half lb. chicken	4	cloves garlic, peeled
3	or 4 stalks celery with leaves	1	small bunch parsley
1	onion, peeled and cut in half	½	cup mushroom stems
		2	cups dry white wine
		1	tsp. salt

Place the chicken in large kettle. Cover with water to within about 3 inches of the rim of pot to allow for wine. Bring to a boil, then lower heat to simmering and skim off the scum that will rise to the surface. When clear, add remaining ingredients and cook over very low heat until chicken is tender.

Remove chicken to a platter and set aside until cool enough to handle.

Remove meat from chicken. Place it in a container, cover and refrigerate until ready to use.

Return chicken bones and less desirable pieces, such as wings and back, to stock and continue to simmer for 4 to 5 hours. As with beef stock, it will take on a shiny appearance when it is done.

Cool, then strain into a large bowl, discarding bones and vegetables. Refrigerate until fat rises to the surface and hardens. Remove and discard fat.

Ladle stock into pint-size Mason jars and refrigerate or freeze until needed (about 40 calories per cup).

QUICK CHICKEN STOCK

2 eight-oz. cans condensed chicken broth	Several sprigs parsley
	A few mushroom stems, trimmed and chopped
2 cups water	
1 cup dry white wine	1 small bay leaf
1 small onion, peeled and sliced	¼ tsp. thyme

Combine ingredients in a heavy saucepan and bring to a boil. Lower heat and simmer gently for about 30 minutes. Strain before using.

Makes about 3 cups of stock (about 40 calories per cup).

SAUCE FOR LEFTOVER COOKED CHICKEN OR TURKEY

Here are two ways to make a really superb but low-calorie sauce for leftover chicken or turkey. Both are easy when you have a flavorful stock on hand as the base.

CURRY SAUCE

1 tbs. butter
1 tbs. curry powder
1½ cups chicken stock, heated
½ cup dry white wine
4 dried apricots, chopped

1 tbs. cornstarch, mixed with 1 tbs. good brandy or water
Salt
Pepper

Melt the butter in a saucepan and stir in curry powder. Add heated chicken stock slowly and blend with curry mixture. When smooth, add wine and apricots. Bring to a boil, then lower heat and simmer until reduced by about half.

Remove apricots with a slotted spoon and transfer to an electric blender. Add about a cup of the hot stock mixture and blend to a purée. Return this to the stock mixture. Blend, stir in cornstarch paste and cook, stirring, until sauce thickens. Season to taste with salt and pepper.

Makes about 1 cup sauce (about 200 calories per cup).

NOTE: For leftover turkey or chicken slices, remove meat from refrigerator and bring to room temperature.

Place slices in a shallow baking dish that can be used for serving and pour sauce over them. Heat briefly in a 400° oven. Sprinkle sauce, if you like, with a little paprika or minced parsley just before serving.

RICH SHERRY-CREAM SAUCE

1½ cups chicken stock	2 tbs. Crème Fraiche
½ cup good quality dry	(see page 102)
sherry	Salt
	Pepper

Combine stock and sherry in a small saucepan. Bring to a full boil, then lower heat and simmer until reduced by about half. Stir a little of the hot liquid into the Crème Fraiche, then stir this back into the liquid and blend until smooth and hot over low heat. Season with salt and pepper.

Makes about 1½ cups sauce (about 170 calories per cup).

Another elegant sauce for leftover turkey is simplicity itself. Bring one cup of chicken stock to a boil, lower heat and simmer until reduced by half. Add 1 tbs. currant jelly and stir over low heat until reduced to a smooth, thick, syrupy sauce. Add turkey slices or chopped turkey and heat briefly.

MUSHROOM SHALLOT SAUCE

2 tbs. butter	1½ cups chicken stock
4 to 6 shallots, peeled and finely minced	2 tsps. cornstarch, mixed to a paste with
4 to 6 large fresh mushrooms, peeled and finely minced	1 tbs. water
	Salt
3 tbs. dry Madeira	Pepper

Melt the butter in a saucepan. In it cook shallots and mushrooms over low heat, stirring frequently, until they are very soft, liquid has evaporated and mixture is very dark. Add Madeira, raise heat slightly and cook for 2 or 3 minutes more. Add stock and simmer until reduced by about one third. Stir in cornstarch paste and continue stirring until mixture thickens. Season with salt and pepper.

Makes about 1 cup of sauce (about 250 calories per cup).

15
About Fish

ABOUT COOKING FISH

Fresh fish is as beautiful to cook as it is to eat. It can make you beautiful too. To overcook it is sacrilegious. All fish and seafood has distinctive and delicate flavor along with health-giving qualities. To overpower fish with an incompatible sauce and too many garnishes is to destroy it. Fish cookery should be simplicity itself; the less you fuss with the cooking the better the results.

Beautiful Buffet
For a Summer Night

Cold Striped Bass
with Mayonnaise Rouge Colle

Cold Green Beans   French Potato
Vinaigrette   Salad
Italian Breadsticks
Dry White Wine

Strawberries
with Cognac and a Light Sprinkling
of Confectioners' Sugar

Black Coffee

A VERY FESTIVE PLATTER
(WONDERFUL FOR A DIET-CONSCIOUS
BUFFET SUPPER)
COLD STRIPED BASS
WITH MAYONNAISE ROUGE COLLÉE

(Basic recipe for poached bass or any other firm white
fish)

2½ qts. water   2 thin slices lemon
 2 cups dry white wine   2 bay leaves
 1 large mild-flavored   8 to 10 peppercorns
    onion, peeled and   1 six- to eight-lb. striped
    sliced   bass, with head and
 1 clove garlic, peeled   tail left on
    and split in half
    (optional)

Combine all ingredients but fish in a fish poacher.
Bring to a boil, then lower heat and simmer very gently
for about 30 minutes. Place fish on poacher rack. The fish
should be barely covered by liquid. If necessary, add a
little additional wine or water. Return liquid to simmering and poach the fish for 8 minutes to the pound. The
water should barely be bubbing.

Off the heat, allow the fish to cool in the liquid for
about 20 minutes. Lift the fish out gently and slide it onto
a double-thick layer of cheesecloth (reserve stock). Remove and discard top skin. Then gently cut the fish open,
and spread each side out flat, leaving bottom intact. Lift
top end of backbone and gently pull it off in one piece.
Then remove as many remaining loose bones as you
neatly can. Lift ends of cheesecloth and use it to help flip
fish back together. Gently press it into original shape.

Use the cheesecloth again to help lift the fish and slide
it onto a serving platter. Cover platter completely with

plastic wrap and refrigerate fish without Mayonnaise while preparing Mayonnaise Rouge Collé. (About 200 calories per serving.)

MAYONNAISE ROUGE COLLÉE

1 tsp. catsup	½ envelope unflavored
2 or 3 dashes red-hot	gelatin
pepper sauce	½ cup reserved fish
¾ cup mayonnaise (see	stock
recipe page 210-11)	

Stir catsup and hot sauce into mayonnaise.

Sprinkle gelatin over stock in a small saucepan and stir over very low heat until dissolved. Stir mixture into mayonnaise.

Chill until slightly thickened before assembling fish platter (about 110 calories per tablespoon).

FISH PLATTER

Cold poached, chilled	1 small jar red caviar
and boned 6 to 8 lb.	2 thinly sliced small
striped bass	cucumbers
(see recipe page 136)	6 to 8 thinly sliced
Mayonnaise collée (see	pimiento-stuffed green
recipe page 137)	olives

Cover fish with a thin, even layer of mayonnaise collée and sprinkle caviar down center. Surround with cucumber slices and top each with an olive slice.

Serves 4 (about 300 calories per serving).

FISH STOCK

2 lbs. fish bones and head	6 or 8 sprigs parsley
1 quart water	1 bay leaf
1 medium mild onion, peeled and chopped	Pinch dried thyme
1 stalk celery with leaves, coarsely chopped	6 to 8 peppercorns
1 clove garlic, peeled and split in half lengthwise, halves flattened with the side of a heavy cleaver	1 to 2 cups dry white wine
	½ tsp. salt

Place fish and bones in a large heavy pot. Add water and bring to a boil. Skim surface until clear.

Add remaining ingredients, lower heat and simmer for about 1 hour. Strain through a fine sieve or a colander lined with cheesecloth. Use to poach any fish or fish fillets.

If desired, can be made ahead. Refrigerate, covered, for use within two or three days. Bring to full boil again before using. Or pour into clean Mason jars, seal and store in freezer for 2 to 3 weeks. To use, place jar in a pan of cold water until sufficiently thawed to pour contents into cooking pot. Bring to boil before using (about 10 calories per cup).

WHITE WINE SAUCE
FOR BROILED, BAKED OR POACHED FISH

1½ cups fish stock	Salt
½ cup dry white wine	Pepper
1 tbs. cornstarch, blended to a paste with 2 tbs. Cognac or good brandy	

Combine stock and wine in a small saucepan and bring to a boil. Lower heat and simmer until reduced by about half. Stir in cornstarch-Cognac paste. Season to taste and stir over low heat until smooth and thick.

Makes about 1 cup of sauce (about 20 calories per cup).

SEAFOOD MARINARA

16 to 18 large shrimp	1 one-lb. can Italian-style tomatoes with basil
2 lobster tails (preferably fresh; if frozen, defrost)	
12 cherrystone clams	½ cup dry white wine
¼ cup olive oil (or, if preferred, vegetable oil)	1 bay leaf
	1 tsp. mixed Italian herbs
2 cloves garlic, peeled and minced	Salt
	Pepper
	¼ cup minced parsley

Split the shells of the shrimp lengthwise down the entire back; devein but do not remove the shells. Rinse and blot dry. Wash the lobster tails and, with a large kitchen knife, cut them crosswise (unshelled) into 1-inch slices. Thoroughly scrub clams under cold running water. Use a steel vegetable brush if you have one, but whatever you use make sure all sand and grit are removed.

Heat the oil in a large heavy stewpot. Add garlic and, over medium heat, sauté until limp. Add shrimp and lobster and cook, stirring gently, for about 2 minutes.

Add tomatoes, wine, bay leaf and herbs. Season lightly with salt, and heavily with black pepper. Bring to a boil, then lower heat and simmer for 2 to 3 minutes, stirring frequently.

Add the clams, cover and continue to cook (fairly high heat now), shaking the pot frequently and stirring occasionally for 10 to 12 minutes or until clams open. (Remove and discard any clams that do not open after 12 minutes of cooking.) Sprinkle with parsley and serve very hot.

4 servings (about 250 calories per serving).

FILLET OF FLOUNDER BAKED IN FOIL

Any firm white fish may be substituted. However, for best flavor, it should be freshly caught.

1 large onion, peeled and chopped	3 tbs. tarragon vinegar
1 clove garlic, peeled and minced	4 tbs. olive oil
½ tsp. mixed Italian herbs	6 flounder fillets
½ tsp. salt	2 large unpeeled tomatoes, sliced
¼ tsp. black pepper	Juice from ½ large lemon
	Lemon wedges

Preheat oven to 425°.

Line a long shallow baking dish with sufficient foil to cover and lightly seal in the fillets.

Combine onion, garlic, herbs, salt, pepper, vinegar and oil. Pour half of mixture in bottom of the foil-lined pan. Arrange fillets on top in single layer. Cover with tomato slices and pour remaining mixture over surface. Sprinkle with lemon juice, then bring foil up and over and, leaving space at top, fold foil together, sealing in fish and "sauce." Bake for 30 to 35 minutes or until fish flakes easily. Check toward the end to avoid overcooking.

Using a spatula, carefully transfer fillets and tomatoes to serving plates and spoon "sauce" over surface. Serve with lemon wedges.

4 servings (about 250 calories per serving).

RAINBOW TROUT SAUTÉ
WITH WINE SAUCE

4 trout about ¾ lb. each, cleaned and ready to cook	½ cup dry white wine
	¼ cup lemon juice, freshly squeezed and strained
Salt	
Pepper	1 tsp. cornstarch, mixed to a paste with 1 tbs. water
1 cup all-purpose flour	
½ cup vegetable oil, or more if needed	
2 tbs. butter	¼ cup minced parsley

Season trout with salt and pepper to taste. Roll trout in flour; shake off excess.

Use a heavy skillet sufficiently large to hold all of the fish in one layer (or sauté two at a time in a smaller skillet, using fresh oil and butter after first two are cooked).

Place skillet over medium heat. Add oil and butter. When butter has melted and oil is hot, add the fish and cook, turning once, until golden brown on each side (about 5 minutes per side) or until fish flakes easily when touched with a fork.

Remove fish to a heated platter. Pour off and discard

cooking oil and butter. Wipe skillet clean with paper toweling. Pour in wine and lemon juice and bring to a boil. Lower heat and add cornstarch paste, stirring until sauce is slightly thickened. Season with a little salt if necessary. Stir in minced parsley, pour over fish and serve at once.

4 servings (about 250 calories per serving).

SATURDAY-NIGHT SPECIAL:
PAULEY'S ISLAND
FISH STEW

This is favorite Saturday-night fare on lovely, unspoiled Pauley's Island just north of Charleston, South Carolina. Many Charlestonians have cottages here and drive up on Friday night and use Saturday's catch to make this wonderfully satisfying fish stew. Informality is the word and most of the guests are barefoot. It's the food that counts, not the fanfare. What makes the stew extra special is that you can enjoy and not repent; the calorie count is way down there.

All you need add for a complete meal is freshly cooked rice, and a good choice for dessert might be sliced peaches with a sprinkling of Cognac or a spoonful of Grand Marnier Sauce.

2 tbs. olive oil
1 large onion, peeled and chopped
2 stalks celery with leaves, coarsely chopped
2 cloves garlic, peeled and minced
1 tsp. saffron threads
1 one-lb. can plum tomatoes
2 large fresh tomatoes, peeled and chopped
1 bay leaf
8 to 10 peppercorns
½ tsp. dried oregano
1 cup dry white wine
1 cup clam juice or use

fish stock (see page 138)
2 cups water
2 lbs. firm-fleshed fish,
   such as striped bass,
   sea bass or carp, cut
   into chunks

2 dozen clams, scrubbed
   and washed well
1 tb. Pernod (optional)
¼ cup finely chopped
   parsley

Place the oil in a large heavy stewpot over medium heat. Add onion, celery and garlic. Cook, stirring, until vegetables are tender. Add saffron threads and stir for 1 to 2 minutes.

Add canned and fresh tomatoes, bay leaf, peppercorns and oregano. Pour in wine, clam juice and water (or wine and fish stock). Bring to a boil, lower heat and simmer, uncovered, for 30 to 40 minutes.

Add the fish and clams. Cover pot, increase heat and boil briskly for about 20 minutes, or until clams have opened. (Remove and discard any that do not open.)

Add Pernod and parsley. Cover and shake pot vigorously to combine ingredients. Serve in soup bowls.

Hot garlic bread (one thick slice per "dieter") could be the luxurious accompaniment to this dish. Despite its richness, it is still calorie low (4 servings about 400 per serving).

STRIPED BASS ITALIAN STYLE

1 four-lb. striped bass, cleaned and left whole	2 cups (canned) Italian cooking sauce
½ cup lemon juice	½ cup dry white wine
Salt	1 lemon, thinly sliced
Pepper	8 to 12 cherrystone clams, washed and scrubbed
1 medium onion, peeled and chopped	
1 clove garlic, peeled and minced	8 large shrimp, back of shells split lengthwise (to devein) but not removed
½ cup parsley, chopped	
1 tsp. mixed Italian herbs	

Preheat oven to 450°.

Slit bass lengthwise down the top of each side. Rub well on each side and inside with lemon juice, salt and pepper.

Place fish in the center of a glass baking dish. Sprinkle over and around it the onion, garlic, parsley and herbs. Combine sauce and wine and pour over and around fish and vegetables.

Top with lemon slices. Cover and place in preheated oven for 25 minutes.

Remove and arrange clams on one side of fish, shrimp on the other. Cover and return to oven. Reduce heat to 375° and continue to bake for another 15 to 20 minutes, or until clams have opened.

Arrange a portion of the fish, two clams and two shrimp on each serving plate. Spoon sauce over all and serve at once.

4 servings (about 350 calories per serving).

Rice is the best accompaniment for this dish. No vegetable is needed as the sauce takes its place.

FEAST FOR A FRIDAY NIGHT

*Tarragon Grilled Fish
with Cucumbers*

Cheese-Stuffed Baked Potatoes

Oranges in Wine

Coffee

TARRAGON GRILLED FISH
WITH CUCUMBERS

6 medium-size cucumbers, peeled and thinly sliced	4 tbs. butter
½ cup tarragon vinegar	¼ cup fresh lemon juice
1 cup ice water	½ tsp. dried tarragon
1 three-and-a-half to four-lb. fish (or two smaller ones), cleaned and split (sea bass, red snapper or white fish)	½ tsp. salt
	Tarragon Mayonnaise

Combine vinegar with 1 cup of ice water and pour over the cucumbers. Cover and refrigerate for about 1 hour before preparing fish. Drain just before using and pat dry.

Preheat broiler.

Place fish, skin side down, in a well-buttered shallow pan.

Melt the butter in a small saucepan. Stir in lemon juice, tarragon and salt. Brush fish with some of the mixture. Place about 3 inches under high broiler flame. Broil for 5 minutes, basting with some of the butter mixture. Turn and broil for a second 5 minutes and baste once more. Test with fork. When fish flakes easily, it is done. Baste again with remaining butter mixture.

Transfer to serving platter. Surround with cucumber slices and cover center of fish with a ribbon of Tarragon Mayonnaise. Serve at once.

Serves 4 (about 800 calories per serving with 1 tb. Tarragon Mayonnaise per serving).

Two tips: Remember to lift broiler rack to about 3 inches below flame level before heating broiler. Fish "weeps" if it's too far from the heat.

And don't overcook. Get fish out of the oven as soon as it's done or it will be dry and unappealing.

TARRAGON MAYONNAISE

1 cup mayonnaise   2 tbs. tarragon vinegar
   (preferably
   homemade)

Blend together just before using (about 100 calories per tablespoon).

16
A Variety of Chicken

DINNER PARTY FOR FOUR

*Red Caviar on Unsalted Water Biscuits
or Homemade Melba Toast*

*French-Style Roast Chicken
with Wine Sauce*

*Stir-Fried Peas with Small
White Onions*

Dry White Wine

*Lemon Sponge Cake with
Puréed Strawberries*

Black Coffee

CLASSIC FRENCH ROAST CHICKEN

This recipe does, indeed, call for butter, but as the resulting sauce is chilled and cleared of all fat before reheating and serving with the chicken calories are reduced, though all butter flavor remains. As with all cooking, the results depend on the ingredients, so try to buy a freshly killed rather than a frozen bird. The taste is far superior.

1 young chicken, about 3 lbs.	1 medium onion, peeled and cut into thick slices
5 tbs. butter	
1 tsp. lemon juice	1 carrot, scraped and cut into thick slices
½ tsp. salt	
Freshly ground black pepper	1 cup chicken stock
	½ cup dry white wine

Preheat oven to 475°.

Wash the chicken and dry well with paper toweling. Cream 2 tbs. of the butter and gradually work in the lemon juice, salt and pepper. Spread this seasoned butter inside the chicken. Melt the remaining butter and spread over the outside of chicken.

Place the chicken on its side on a rack in shallow roasting pan. Roast for 15 minutes, then, using a wooden spoon, turn and roast the opposite side for 15 minutes.

Put the chicken on its back and lower the oven heat to 400°. Add the sliced onions and carrots to the roasting pan under the rack along with ½ cup of the stock. Baste the chicken and roast for about 40 minutes longer. To test for doneness lift the chicken with a wooden spoon. If the juices that run out are clear, the bird is done. Remove to a platter and keep warm.

Strain the accumulated liquid into a small saucepan and place in the freezer until fat has risen and congealed. Remove and discard fat. Combine liquid with remaining stock and wine. Bring to a boil and cook over medium heat until reduced by half. Serve with sliced roast chicken.

Chicken roasted in this manner has a wonderful crisp

skin, but it's moist and tender within. Served hot with
sauce, or cold with either a fruit or vegetable salad, it is
superb eating.

Serves 4 (about 375 calories per serving).

SUMMER SUNDAY LUNCH

Jellied Chicken Loaf
with Homemade Mayonnaise

Picked Beets   *Cucumber Fingers*
Italian Breadsticks

Cottage Cheese Peach "Ice Cream"

Black Coffee

JELLIED CHICKEN LOAF

1 envelope unflavored
  gelatin
2 tbs. cold water
1½ cups homemade
  chicken stock (see
  page 130)
½ tsp. salt
  Mayonnaise

2 cups diced cooked
  chicken
½ cup diced celery
1 tsp. grated onion
½ cup sliced pimiento-
  stuffed olives
  Lettuce leaves

Soften gelatin in cold water. Heat chicken stock to
simmering in a small saucepan and dissolve gelatin in
hot stock. Add salt and pour into a 10-inch-long loaf pan
that has been lightly greased with mayonnaise. Chill
until slightly thickened, then add chicken, celery, onion
and olives. When prepared this way, the chicken and
other ingredients remain evenly distributed, instead of

sinking to the bottom of the gelatin mixture. When firm, unmold onto a lettuce-lined platter and serve with homemade mayonnaise (see recipe page 210).
Serves six (128 calories per serving).

NOTE: If not using homemade chicken stock that has already thickened naturally, use 2 envelopes of gelatin.

CURRY DINNER FOR SIX

Cold Broccoli Vinaigrette

Chicken Curry
Chutney   Shredded Coconut
Minced Parsley

(The traditional, but not necessary, chopped peanuts are omitted for calorie-conscious diners)

Freshly Cooked White Rice

Dry White Wine

*Fresh Strawberries
with Grand Marnier*

Black Coffee

CHICKEN CURRY

1 tbs. butter	1 tbs. flour
1 large onion, peeled and finely minced	2 tbs. curry powder
	3 cups chicken stock
2 large tart apples, peeled, cored and chopped	3 cups diced cooked chicken

Melt the butter in a large heavy saucepan over very low heat. Add minced onion and chopped apple and cook until onions are very soft and apple has been reduced to a pulp. Do not allow to brown. Add flour and continue to cook for 1 to 2 minutes. Add curry powder and stock. Blend and allow to cook for 20 to 30 minutes, still over low heat, until sauce thickens. (May be prepared ahead to this point.) Add diced chicken and cook until chicken is thoroughly hot. Serve over freshly cooked rice with suggested accompaniments (see page 150).

Serves 6 (about 235 calories per serving).

ROCK CORNISH HENS IN
WHITE WINE SAUCE

4 rock cornish game hens	1 bay leaf
2 tbs. unsalted butter	1 to 2 tbs. arrowroot
6 to 8 shallots, peeled and minced	Madeira
	Salt
	Pepper
2 cups dry white wine	Lemon juice
4 cups chicken stock (or more depending on size of hens)	¼ to ½ cup minced parsley

If hens are frozen, have your butcher thaw them and cut each in half.

Preheat oven to 400°.

Arrange hens, skin side up, side by side, in a roasting pan. Place in preheated oven and roast, uncovered, until well browned, about 15 minutes. Turn and roast, skin side down, for about 10 minutes more, then roast skin side up again for a final 5 minutes. Remove pan from oven. Remove hens and set aside.

Pour off rendered fat from pan and return birds to it, skin side up. Set aside.

Melt butter in a small saucepan, add shallots and sauté over low heat until very soft. Pour in wine, raise heat and cook, stirring often, until reduced by half, then pour over hens in roasting pan. Add sufficient chicken stock so hens are barely covered. Add bay leaf. Cover and place in oven (heat lowered to 350°) until hens are very tender, about 30 minutes.

Remove hens to serving platter. On top of stove, over high heat, stir cooking liquid to reduce a little and intensify flavor. Remove and discard bay leaf. Blend arrowroot with a little Madeira to make a paste. Off the heat, stir this into the reduced cooking liquid, then cook, stirring to a smooth thick sauce. Taste and season with salt and pepper and, if desired, a little lemon juice. Return hens to sauce and heat thoroughly. Sprinkle with parsley just before serving.

Serves 8 (about 400 calories per serving).

The 8 halves of cornish hens will, of course give you 8 portions. One-half hen makes an ample serving when accompanied by rice and a broiled fresh peach half.

If it's a party, you might start this meal with a first-course vegetable. Steamed fresh asparagus or tomatoes vinaigrette are both good choices.

CHICKEN,
MEXICAN STYLE

4 chicken legs and
4 chicken thighs
3 stalks celery, chopped
1 medium onion, peeled
   and chopped
1 (small can) Jalapeño
   chilies, chopped
3 cloves garlic, peeled
   and minced
½ cup dry white wine

½ tsp. salt
½ tsp. freshly ground
   black pepper
1 small can Tomatillos
   (Mexican Green
   Tomatoes)
½ cup plain yogurt
   Fresh coriander or
   parsley, minced

Preheat oven to 350°.

Arrange chicken legs and thighs, skin side up, not touching, in a single layer in a shallow baking dish. Place in preheated oven and bake for 30 minutes.

Remove from oven. Blot chicken pieces with paper toweling to remove rendered fat. Pour off and discard rendered fat from baking dish and wipe it clean with paper toweling.

Combine celery, onion, chilies and garlic and cover bottom of baking dish with the mixture. Arrange chicken pieces on top. Pour wine over them and sprinkle with salt and pepper. Cover and seal dish with foil and return it to the oven to bake for a second 30 minutes.

Remove chicken pieces to a serving platter and keep warm.

Transfer vegetables and cooking liquid from baking dish to an electric blender. Add Tomatillos and blend to a purée. Pour into a hevy saucepan and add yogurt. Heat, stirring, to "steaming" hot (do not allow to boil.) Pour over chicken pieces and sprinkle with coriander or parsley.

Serves 4 (about 300 calories per serving).

Serve with rice.

17
The New Ways to Cook Meat

SUPPER FOR A SUMMER NIGHT

*Cold Beef Slices
with Yogurt-Horseradish Sauce*

*Hot Boiled New Potatoes
(Skin Left On)*

*Tomato Slices Vinaigrette
with Chopped Parsley*

Dry Red Wine

Fresh Peaches in Wine

Black Coffee

SUPPER FOR A SUMMER NIGHT

A classic pot roast can be truly a gourmet dish. What's more it is equally good hot or cold and any leftovers are much too delectable to be called leftovers. Serve re-heated in a wine-and-stock sauce or cold with a variety of sauces such as Yogurt-Horseradish Sauce (see page 157)or—a sweet indulgence—a small amount of Cumber-land Sauce (page 157).

1 tbs. salad oil	5 cups beef stock
1 four- to five-lb. boneless pot roast (bottom round is first choice)	2 cups dry red wine
	1 carrot, scraped and cut into chunks
2 or 3 beef marrow bones	1 onion, peeled and quartered
	3 cloves garlic, peeled

Preheat oven to 400°.

Cover the bottom of a large 6- to 8-quart pot with a thin film of oil. Add meat and bones. Place in preheated oven for about 20 minutes, or until well browned. Browning the meat in this manner uses far less fat and that is our goal.

Place pot on top of stove. Add stock, wine, vegetables and garlic. Bring to a boil, then lower heat to barely simmering. Simmer, partially covered, for 2 to 3 hours, or until meat is tender. Do not pierce meat to determine tenderness as it will lose juices and be dry and tasteless if allowed to cook after piercing. Press with a wooden spoon instead. If liquid is not sufficient to cover meat, turn several times during cooking, using two wooden spoons to avoid piercing meat. If necessary add another cup of stock or, if you have to, a cup or two of cold water. This should not be needed, however, if cooking is done over very low heat.

When the roast is tender, remove it to a platter. Cover with plastic wrap and, unless you are planning to serve it the same day, refrigerate until ready to reheat. Otherwise leave at room temperature until ready to reheat in sauce.

Strain cooking liquid into a saucepan, discarding vegetables and bones, and place in freezer for an hour or two until fat rises to the surface and congeals. Remove and discard fat.

When ready to serve, place meat in cooking liquid over medium heat for about 20 minutes. Remove meat and reduce liquid over high heat to about half. Serve meat sliced and accompanied by sauce with steamed carrots and boiled small white onions.

1 four-oz. serving about 400 calories.

Leftover slices may be reheated in sauce or served cold with any of the following sauces. If extra slices are to be stored in the refrigerator, cover with cooking liquid to prevent drying.

YOGURT-HORSERADISH SAUCE

½ cup yogurt   1 tsp. grated onion
3 tbs. bottled   Dash of Tabasco
    horseradish

Combine all ingredients and blend well. Keep refrigerated until ready to use.

Serves 4 (about 20 calories per serving).

CUMBERLAND SAUCE

½ cup currant jelly   1 tsp. grated onion
½ cup bottled   (optional)
    horseradish

Combine ingredients and chill until ready to serve.
4 servings (about 120 calories per serving).

APRICOT PORT WINE SAUCE

8 ozs. dried apricots	2 tsps. curry powder
½ cup port wine	½ cup plain yogurt

Place apricots in a medium saucepan and add only enough water to cover them. Cook over low heat until they are very soft and all liquid has been absorbed. Add port and stir in curry powder. Continue to cook until liquid has again been absorbed. Mash to a pulp or purée in electric blender. Refrigerate until chilled. Stir in yogurt.

This makes an excellent sauce for cold meat.

Makes about 4 servings (about 75 calories per serving).

BARBECUED POT ROAST

This is a wonderfully spicy hot pot roast that is not just good on the first serving but also makes wonderful leftovers. Try cold slices with Green Beans Vinaigrette, or with French Potato Salad (see recipe page 208).

Like all the pot roast and stew recipes in this book this one calls for chilling and removing all fat before serving, so the calorie count per slice is within a dieter's menu limits.

1 four-lb. pot roast of beef	2 tbs. tomato paste
1 tbs. salad oil	2 cups water
2 cups sliced onions	½ cup chili sauce
2 cloves of garlic, minced	½ cup apple cider vinegar
1 tsp. salt	2 tbs. Worcestershire sauce
1 one-lb. can of tomatoes	1 tbs. chili powder

Preheat oven to 400°.

Have the butcher trim the fat from the roast. Cover the bottom of a deep heavy pot with a thin film of oil and brown the meat in the preheated oven.

Transfer to the top of the stove. Remove meat and set aside. Add the onions and garlic to the pot and cook over low heat until soft but not brown. Return meat to pot. Add salt, tomatoes, tomato paste and water. Simmer over medium heat for about 2 hours or until meat begins to be tender. It should not boil. Add chili sauce, vinegar, Worcestershire sauce and chili powder. Blend well into cooking liquid and cook for 1 hour longer.

Remove meat to a platter, cover with plastic wrap and refrigerate until ready to reheat. Cover pot and refrigerate sauce until fat has hardened and risen to the surface. This takes at least 4 hours. Remove and discard fat. Slice meat and reheat in the sauce over low heat before serving. (About 400 calories per each 4 oz. serving.)

SLICED RUMP ROAST
WITH ORANGES

Here is another lean cut of meat that's a good calorie cutter. If it is prime grade, steaks cut from it may be broiled or it may be left in one 4- to 5-lb. triangular piece and roasted. If it is choice grade, however—and in most markets it is—it is better when braised as a pot roast. Like other less-tender cuts of beef, a rump roast has superb flavor. It also has the added plus of being close-grained meat and is firm in texture so that it slices easily.

1 four- to four-and-a-
   half-lb. boneless rump
   of beef
1 cup dry red wine
2 cups beef stock (see
   page 127-29)
   Water
2 tsps. salt
1 large onion, peeled
   and quartered

3 cloves garlic
1 bay leaf
1 tsp. coriander seeds,
   slightly crushed
½ cup fresh orange juice
2 seedless oranges,
   peeled and sliced

Preheat oven to 500°.

Bring beef to room temperature. Place on a rack in a shallow roasting pan in preheated oven, and roast until browned, about 15 minutes.

Transfer browned meat to a heavy pot (one with a tight-fitting lid). Add wine, stock and sufficient water to cover. Add salt and bring to a full boil. Skim surface until liquid is clear, then add onion, garlic, bay leaf and coriander seeds. Reduce heat and simmer gently until meat is tender, about 2 hours. Remove from heat and let stand for about 1 hour.

Remove meat from liquid and let stand for about 15 minutes, then slice thin and arrange slices, overlapping slightly, in a long shallow baking dish. Boil cooking liquid down to about half, strain, add orange juice and pour over meat. Cover dish and seal with foil. Refrigerate up to 24 hours.

Remove and discard any fat on surface of meat and sauce. Place orange slices over meat and liquid in baking dish. Reheat in a 375° oven and serve from the dish. Or drain and arrange orange slices over meat on serving platter.

8 to 10 servings (about 400 calories per serving).

A CLASSIC SPRING DINNER

Roast Leg of Lamb

Mint Jelly
(small serving)
Boiled Tiny New Potatoes in Their Jackets

Fresh Asparagus

Wine—Red Bordeaux

Stewed Rhubarb

Black Coffee

SUNDAY NIGHT COLD SUPPER

Cold Sliced Roast Lamb

Salsa Fria

French Potato Salad

Lime Mousse

Black Coffee

ROAST LEG OF LAMB
IN THE GREEK MANNER

Leg of lamb, though certainly not cheap, is a good buy as there is little waste. It is also lower in calories than beef. This marinated roast is delicious hot or cold and any remaining scraps can be ground and spread on extra-thin toast to make an unusual hors d'oeuvre.

1	six- to seven-lb. leg of lamb	1	tsp. mixed Italian herbs
½	cup fresh lemon juice	¼	cup minced parsley
½	cup fresh orange juice	2	tsps. salt
½	cup dry white wine	2	tsps. freshly ground black pepper
¼	cup salad oil Grated peel of 1 lemon		
4	cloves of garlic, peeled and finely minced		

Place the leg of lamb in a long non-metal pan; a glass baking dish is ideal. Combine all remaining ingredients in a non-metal bowl. Allow lamb and marinade to come to room temperature, stirring the marinade frequently to blend flavors.

Pour marinade over lamb and allow to stand for 3 to 4 hours, basting frequently.

Preheat oven to 400°. Turn lamb fat side up and score in several places with a sharp knife. Spoon marinade over lamb and roast for about 14 minutes to the pound basting frequently with marinade and pan juices. If you don't like your lamb slightly pink, roast for 18 minutes to the lb. Or the lamb may be grilled over charcoal, using a meat thermometer to determine doneness. It should register 150 degrees when inserted in thickest part of the meat.

Remove lamb to carving platter and allow to stand for 10 to 15 minutes. Discard pan juice as it will be too greasy to be enjoyed.

About 215 calories per 4 oz. serving.

Cold leftover lamb makes a star repeat performance when served with this inspired hot-pepper sauce.

SALSA FRIA

4 tomatoes, peeled, seeded and chopped	1 tbs. salad oil
½ cup finely minced green onion	1½ tbs. red wine vinegar
1 green pepper, seeded, white removed, finely chopped	¼ tsp. salt
	¼ tsp. fresh black pepper
2 cloves garlic, peeled and minced	3 dried red chilies, crushed
1 four-oz. can Mexican chilies, finely chopped	Pinch of ground cumin

Mix all ingredients together in a non-metal bowl and refrigerate for several hours before serving. Will keep for a week if kept cold.

Makes about 3 cups relish (about 50 calories per ½ cup serving).

VEAL CUTLETS MARSALA

Veal, having very little fat, is an ideal choice for the dieter when meat is what is wanted. Try this easy, quick recipe for Veal Cutlets in Marsala wine. Add small boiled new potatoes in their jackets and perhaps a serving of fresh asparagus.

Dessert could be fruit and cheese in the Italian manner, or the Orange Champagne Ring (see page 221).

½ cup flour	2 tbs. butter
1 tsp. salt	2 tbs. vegetable oil
1 tsp. freshly ground black pepper	½ cup Marsala
1½ lbs. of veal cutlet, cut into slices then pounded as thin as possible	

Mix together the flour, salt and pepper. Dip cutlets in seasoned flour, shake off excess. Melt butter with the oil in a large heavy skillet and brown the cutlets in the mixture. Remove cutlets to a heated platter. Drain any remaining oil from skillet and wipe dry with paper toweling. Return cutlets to skillet, add Marsala and cook over medium heat for about 5 minutes.

Serves 4 to 6 (4 servings, about 350 calories per serving; 6 servings, 290 calories per serving).

VEAL MARENGO

2 tbs. salad oil	1 tbs. flour
2 lbs. boneless leg or rump of veal, cut into 2-in. cubes	½ tsp. salt
	1 tsp. thyme fresh or dried
1 tbs. butter	1 cup dry red wine
1 tsp. vegetable oil	2 cups fat-free beef stock
¾ cup finely chopped purple onion	
½ cup finely chopped green onion	3 fresh tomatoes, peeled and chopped or 1 one-lb. can tomatoes, drained
3 cloves garlic, minced	

Peel of ½ lemon cut	1 tbs. tomato paste
into strips	½ lb. fresh mushrooms,
1 bay leaf	trimmed and sliced

Preheat oven to 400°.

Barely cover the bottom of a large pot with a thin film of salad oil. Add the meat and place in preheated oven to brown. This should take about 15 minutes. Turn two or three times to brown evenly. Meanwhile melt the butter in a small saucepan over very low heat and sauté the onions and garlic until soft but not brown.

Remove the pot containing the browned meat to the top of the stove and sprinkle the contents with flour, salt and thyme. Turn to coat each piece evenly and cook over low heat for 2 or 3 minutes.

Add the sautéed onions, garlic, wine, stock, tomatoes, lemon peel and bay leaf. Bring to a boil, then lower heat to simmering. Cover and cook for about 45 minutes.

Stir in tomato paste. Add the mushrooms and continue to cook for another 15 minutes, or until meat is tender.

Cool the Marengo, then place it in the refrigerator until fat has congealed and risen to the surface. Remove and discard fat. Reheat Marengo slowly until very hot. Serve with one or two small slices of crusty French bread.

Serves 4 to 6 (4 servings about 525 calories per serving; 6 servings about 395 calories per serving).

VEAL STROGANOFF

2 tbs. all-purpose flour	1 medium-size onion,
1 tsp. salt	peeled and chopped
½ tsp. pepper	½ cup dry white wine
1½ lbs. lean veal, very	½ cup fat-free chicken
thinly sliced and cut	stock
into 1-inch strips	½ tsp. prepared mustard
1 tbs. vegetable oil	1 tbs. tomato paste
1 tbs. butter	½ cup yogurt
2 tbs. good quality	
brandy	

Put flour, salt and pepper in a plastic bag. Add veal pieces. Shake to coat veal evenly. Remove from bag and shake off excess flavor.

Combine oil and butter in a large, heavy skillet over high heat. When butter melts, add veal and brown quickly. Add brandy, ignite with a kitchen match, and shake pan over heat until flame subsides. Add onion and stir-fry for 1 minute. Add wine and stock. Stir in mustard and tomato paste. Bring to boiling, lower heat, cover and simmer for about 15 minutes or until meat is tender.

Stir in yogurt and cook, stirring, for a few minutes to heat through (do not allow to boil after adding yogurt).

Serve over hot cooked noodles.

Serves six (about 195 calories per serving).

VEAL RAGOUT

2 lbs. boneless leg of
   veal, fat-trimmed and
   cut into cubes
2 tbs. vegetable oil
1 tsp. salt
½ tsp. pepper
1 tsp. sugar
2 cups fat-free chicken
   stock
1 cup tomato juice
1 clove garlic, peeled
   Pinch thyme,
   crumbled

1 bay leaf
1 lb. carrots, scraped
   and cut into 1-inch
   pieces
½ lb. very small white
   onions, peeled
1 lb. fresh (or if you
   must 1 ten-oz. package
   frozen) green beans
3 tbs. all-purpose flour
½ cup water

In a large heavy pot brown veal cubes well in oil over medium heat. Drain off oil. Sprinkle meat with salt, pepper and sugar. Stir over heat until sugar has dissolved. Add stock, tomato juice, garlic, thyme and bay leaf. Bring to boiling, lower heat, partially cover pot and simmer meat until tender, about 1 hour. Remove from heat. Remove and discard bay leaf and garlic. Refrigerate for several hours or overnight.

About 45 minutes before serving time, remove all congealed fat from ragout. Heat to boiling and add carrots and onions. Cover and simmer for about 20 minutes, or until vegetables are almost tender. Add green beans and simmer until all vegetables are tender.

Combine flour and water and mix to a paste. Stir into simmering ragout. Cook, stirring constantly, until sauce thickens.

6 servings (about 300 calories per serving).

NOTE: Lean leg of lamb may be substituted for veal.

VEAL CURRY

1½ cups fat-free chicken
    stock
½ cup dry white wine
1 medium-size onion,
    peeled and chopped
3 or 4 celery stalks,
    chopped
½ small green pepper,
    chopped fine (seeded,
    white membrane
    removed before
    chopping)

1 clove garlic, peeled
    and minced (optional)
1 large or 2 small crisp
    tart apples, peeled,
    cored and chopped
½ tsp. salt
1 tbs. curry powder
3 cups cubed lean
    cooked veal
1 tbs. cornstarch
¼ cup water
½ cup yogurt

Combine stock, wine, onion, celery, green pepper, garlic, and apples, in a large saucepan. Bring to a full boil, lower heat and simmer until vegetables are tender. Add salt, curry powder and veal. Simmer for about 5 minutes to blend flavors.

Combine cornstarch and water and mix to a paste. Stir into simmering curry. Cook, stirring until thickened. Stir in yogurt and blend until smooth and hot, do not allow to boil after adding yogurt.

6 servings (about 300 calories per serving).

ORGAN MEATS

Many Americans overlook organ meats, often because creative ways to cook them are unknown, or perhaps because the automatic reaction to meat is steak, roast beef or hamburger. But organ meats can be fabulously great-tasting and it's the understatement of the year to say they are wonderfully good for you, not to mention being the lowest-calorie meat you can buy. Rich in the B vitamins, iron and other minerals, organ meats are great "anti-stress" foods. Nutritionists and doctors have known for years that organ meats will not only give you fast "pickup" but great energy, steady nerves and stamina. Since they are so low in calories you can "afford" a rich-tasting sauce, plus a serving of rice or potatoes and still stay far below the calorie count of a steak. Furthermore organ meats can often slenderize your budget. Lamb kidneys are usually quite inexpensive and they make a fantastically good dish in Sauce Bordelaise. Since the total calorie count is low, even with the butter and small amount of Crème Fraiche, you can serve them over a small helping of freshly cooked rice and still stay low on the calorie count.

Or try the recipe (page 170) for Sautéed Calves Liver. Don't say you don't like liver until you try it properly seasoned. No, it does not require bacon as an accompaniment, not when you serve it with Cumberland Sauce (page 157). Naturally a baked potato is the perfect "go with."

As for sweetbreads, they are such a delicacy you will probably reserve them for a festive dinner party once you have tried them A la Marchand du Vin.

As with all good food, organ meats are an acquired taste, but a sophisticated palate is one of the great secrets of successful *pleasant* dieting for a slim, trim body and a beautiful glow of health. It is also the secret of staying with a diet not for a few brief weeks but for life, and for a lifetime of beauty and health.

CALVES LIVER CUMBERLAND

½ lb. calves liver	¼ cup minced shallots
Flour	½ cup dry red wine
Salt	1 tsp. Worcestershire
Pepper	sauce
¼ cup vegetable oil	½ tsp. Dijon mustard
2 tbs. butter	2 tsps. tart currant jelly

Have your butcher slice the liver as thinly as possible. He may resist, saying liver is impossible to slice thin, but if you tell him to chill the liver until it is firm—almost frozen—it will cut nicely into 6 to 8 slices. You can, of course, buy the liver in one piece and do the slicing yourself, but the butcher can, if he will, do a better job with his professional knife on his cutting board.

Dip each slice of liver in flour that has been mixed with a goodly amount of pepper and some salt. Press each slice into the flour so it is completely coated, but shake off all possible excess.

Heat the oil with 1 tbs. of the butter in a large heavy skillet over medium heat. In it quickly brown each slice of liver on both sides. Don't crowd skillet. Brown a few pieces at a time and remove them as soon as browned to a double thickness of paper toweling to drain. (Keep in a single layer.) Blot with more paper toweling to take up all possible cooking oil.

When all slices are browned, pour off and discard all cooking oil from skillet. Add remaining butter and place the skillet over low heat. Add the shallots and sauté until limp. Increase heat. Add wine, Worcestershire, mustard and jelly. Stir until jelly has dissolved.

Return liver slices to skillet and cook, spooning sauce over them, until they are glazed and almost all sauce is absorbed.

Serve very hot with any remaining sauce spooned over meat.

Serves 2 (about 550 calories per serving).

LAMB KIDNEYS BORDELAISE

1 lb. lamb kidneys	½ cup red Bordeaux
2 tbs. butter	1 tbs. Crème Fraiche
½ cup finely minced	(see page 102)
green onion	
2 cups fat-free beef	
stock	

Preheat oven to 350°.

Cut kidneys in small cubes and cut out hard center core. Arrange in a baking casserole with 1 tbs. of the butter and place in preheated oven for about 15 minutes, turning once or twice to coat with butter. Meanwhile melt the remaining butter in a small saucepan and sauté the onion until limp but not brown. Add the stock and wine, blend well. Stir in the Crème Fraiche and blend again. Bring to a simmer and beat with a wire whisk until very smooth. Pour over kidneys in casserole, cover with foil and return to oven. Bake for 30 to 40 minutes, or until kidneys are tender.

Serves 4 (about 200 calories per serving).

RIS DE VEAU À LA MARCHAND DU VIN
(SWEETBREADS IN WINE MERCHANTS' SAUCE)

This is a fabulous dish. You could serve it to a king. It has a luxurious taste unmatched this side of Paris. Fortunately it is extremely low in calories while wonderfully rich in protein, vitamins and minerals, including iron. Since the calorie count of this dish is so low per serving, you can afford to have it over a small portion of freshly cooked rice.

3	pairs of sweetbreads	1	cup dry red wine
2	tbs. lemon juice	12	mushroom caps
2	tbs. butter		(optional)
3	tbs. flour		
½	tsp. salt		
3	cups strong fat-free homemade beef stock (see page 127-29)		

Place the sweetbreads in a large saucepan, preferably non-metal. Cover with cold water, add lemon juice and bring to a boil over high heat. Lower heat to simmering and cook 25 to 30 minutes. Remove from heat, drain and immediately plunge sweetbreads into a bowl of ice water. Add some extra ice cubes to cool them quickly. Refrigerate for at least one hour.

Drain and break the sweetbreads into small pieces. Remove connecting tissue, tubes and membrane-like thin covering. Place sweetbread pieces in long shallow pan such as a glass baking dish. Cover with plastic wrap and weigh down. Use 2 heavy cans, clay tiles or even your iron. Refrigerate again for an additional hour.

Melt the butter in a heavy skillet over medium heat. Combine flour and salt and lightly coat sweetbreads with the mixture. Brown gently in the melted butter. Transfer the sweetbreads to a shallow oven-proof casserole. Add the stock and wine to the skillet and cook over medium heat until reduced to half. Pour over sweetbreads and bake in a 335° oven for 25 to 30 minutes. Serve over freshly cooked rice.

Serves 6 (about 250 calories per serving).

BROILED, MARINATED
CALVES LIVER TERIYAKI

1 lb. calves liver, very thinly sliced (See recipe for Calves Liver Cumberland (p. 170), for slicing directions)
1 tsp. ground ginger, or finely minced fresh or canned ginger root

2 cloves garlic, peeled and cut in half lengthwise
1 tbs. sugar
½ cup dry sherry
½ cup soy sauce
Flour
Vegetable oil

Place liver slices in a long shallow non-metal baking dish. Sprinkle with ginger, garlic and sugar and pour over them the sherry and soy sauce. Let stand at room temperature for about 1 hour, turning the slices occasionally in the marinade.

Drain, reserving marinade, and dredge liver slices with flour, pressing flour into meat, then shaking off excess flour.

Cover the bottom of a large heavy skillet with oil and heat almost to smoking. In it brown each liver slice quickly on both sides. Drain on paper toweling. Strain marinade and pour into 4 small bowls.

Arrange liver slices on individual plates over just-cooked fluffy white rice. Serve a bowl of marinade as dipping sauce with each serving of liver.

4 servings (about 500 calories per serving).

BEEF TONGUE
WITH GREMOLATA MUSTARD

A great dieter's choice. Lean and delicious, simply boiled and served with mustard and, since it is so calorie low, perhaps a bit of currant jelly, Cumberland Sauce (see recipe page 157) or chutney.

A beef tongue can vary in weight from 3 to 4 lbs., give or take a few ounces, mostly due to the way it is trimmed. Large ones include the bone and gristle which must be removed and discarded, so that, larger or smaller, a beef tongue will end up with about the same amount of servings.

1	three- to four-lb. beef tongue	1	bay leaf
1	large onion, peeled	8	to 10 peppercorns
2	cloves garlic, peeled and split lengthwise	1	tsp. salt
2	or 3 celery stalks with leaves		Gremolata mustard (optional)
			Currant jelly (optional)

BOILED BEEF TONGUE

Place tongue in a large heavy pot and cover completely with water. Add the onion, garlic, celery, bay leaf, peppercorns and salt. Bring to a boil, skim surface until clear and simmer over low heat from 2 to 3 hours. Drain and let stand at room temperature until sufficiently cool to remove skin and, if not already removed by the butcher, the gristle, bones and fat portion at large end of tongue. Slice and serve at room temperature. Or place slices in a long shallow baking dish and cover with cooking liquid. Cover dish and refrigerate until ready to serve. Drain before serving and, if desired, spread with plain or Gremolata Mustard.

Slices, chilled or at room temperature, may, if desired, be accompanied by a bit of currant jelly.

3 medium slices about 175 calories.

GREMOLATA MUSTARD

1 clove garlic, peeled
   and chopped
2 tbs. grated lemon rind
½ cup minced parsley

½ cup Dijon style
   mustard (more if
   desired)

Combine and mix well. Serve in a sauce bowl as an accompaniment to any cold meat (about 25 calories per tbs.).

18
Three Great Ways
with Eggs

BAKED EGGS

BASIC RECIPE:

½ cup milk   Salt
4 eggs   Pepper

Preheat oven to 350°.

Butter 4 small custard cups very lightly. Spoon 2 tbs. milk into each.

Break each egg into a cup, then slide it into a prepared custard cup. Sprinkle with salt and pepper. Cover cup and seal with foil.

Bake in preheated oven for 10 minutes or until eggs are done to your taste (about 95 calories per serving).

VARIATIONS:

Sprinkle egg before baking with grated Swiss cheese.
Instead of milk, cover the bottom of each custard cup

177

with chopped, well-drained cooked spinach. Sprinkle eggs lightly with Parmesan cheese.

Before baking spoon 1 tbs. heavy cream over each egg and sprinkle with minced chives. Or, instead of cream, spoon over eggs 1 tbs. chili sauce.

Or cover bottom of each custard cup with a slice of dried chipped beef, add egg and a few dashes of Worcestershire.

Or instead of milk use Pepperide Mix.

PEPPERIDE MIX

2 tbs. olive oil
1 small onion, peeled and minced
½ small green pepper, seeded, white fiber removed, minced

1 large unpeeled fresh tomato, chopped
¼ tsp. black pepper
¼ tsp. salt
Dash Tabasco

Heat oil in a small skillet. In it sauté onion and pepper until very soft. Add chopped tomato and cook, chopping it still further as it cooks with the tip of a spatula. When reduced to a thick sauce, season with pepper, salt and Tabasco (adds about 100 calories per serving to baked eggs).

STUFFED PINK PICKLED EGGS

6 eggs	½ cup cottage cheese
½ cup beet juice from canned beets	1 tsp. mustard
	1 tbs. mayonnaise
¾ cup apple cider vinegar	¼ cup finely minced, well-drained (canned) beets
¼ cup sugar	
1 tbs. mixed pickling spices	2 tbs. finely minced sweet mixed pickle

Bring eggs to room temperature. Cover with water in a large saucepan. Bring to a full boil. Lower heat and simmer for 20 minutes or until hard-cooked. (Do not boil.) Cool eggs under cold running water. Crack shells, and let stand for a few minutes in cold water (shells will slip off easily). Shell and place in a large bowl.

Combine beet juice, vinegar, sugar and pickling spices in a medium saucepan and bring to a boil. Pour over eggs. Let stand about 1 hour, turning often, until whites are tinted an even pink. Drain.

Slice each egg in half and scoop yolks into a mixing bowl. Add remaining ingredients and blend well. Stuff whites with mixture. Refrigerate, covered, until ready to serve.

Serves 6 (about 175 calories per serving).

EGGS FLORENTINE

2 tbs. butter	2 cups chopped, well-drained cooked spinach
2 tbs. flour	
½ tsp. salt	
1½ cups fat-free chicken stock, heated	6 hard-cooked eggs, shelled and sliced
4 tbs. grated Swiss cheese	

Melt the butter in a saucepan and stir in the flour and salt. Cook, stirring, over low heat, for several minutes. Add the heated stock and continue to cook, stirring rapidly, until sauce is thick and smooth.

Stir in cheese. When melted, remove sauce from heat.

Arrange 2 layers each of spinach and egg slices in a shallow 6-cup baking dish. Pour the sauce over.

Bake in preheated 350° oven for about 30 minutes or until bubbly hot.

Serves 6 (about 170 calories per serving).

19
Vegetable Cookery

VEGETABLES

Once you are aware of the nutritional value of fresh vegetables and the happy fact that they are calorie low—forget it and go on to remember how very good they can taste. It's not too late in our culinary history to start serving hot or cold vegetables as a first course, as do the Italians, or even as a second course after a meat or fish entrée in the manner of France. And there are good reasons we should. Vegetables provide more good food for less calories, besides making for a more interesting and satisfying meal.

There is no reason—just because you are on a calorie-restricted diet—to cook vegetables a minute or two in a small amount of water, then serve them unbuttered, unsalted and flavorless, in a half-cooked, half-raw state. Nor is it necessary to overcook and over-sauce them to the point where their naturally sweet, garden-fresh flavor is destroyed along with all of their good-for-you qualities.

Vegetable cookery should be given as much thought as any other part of the meal—or perhaps more. Good vegetable cookery is really a simple affair, rather a matter of timing than anything else.

Frozen vegetables are blanched before being packaged; that is, plunged briefly into boiling water, then into cold water to stop their cooking. Thus much flavor and nutrients are lost.

If you must use frozen vegetables they should be wholly, or at least partially, defrosted before being cooked, in order to retain remaining nutrients as well as flavor. Frozen peas, still cold, but thoroughly defrosted, need be heated only briefly in a little homemade chicken stock, seasoned with salt and pepper and served without further ado. Cooking them frozen in plain water for a longer period will only destroy what little character they have. Frozen spinach should be treated similarly.

Most other frozen vegetables require a bit more time, but, if defrosted, they can be brought to a boil in a little stock, covered and cooked over medium heat until barely tender. Then any liquid that remains in the pan should be boiled away rapidly, with the pan uncovered and shaken constantly to keep the vegetables from sticking. This way nutrients released into the stock during cooking will be returned to the vegetables, and the good rich stock flavor will be absorbed.

BRAISED VEGETABLES

Onions, carrots, turnips, celery—all inexpensive vegetables, take particularly well to braising—that is, cooking—or, more literally, steaming—in flavorful stock. Moreover, they needn't be rushed to the table the minute they are cooked. They may be kept warm for a reasonable time, or, when cold, reheated, even a day later without loss of nutrients or flavor.

BRAISED CARROTS, CALIFORNIA STYLE

½ cup clear fat-free
 chicken stock
¼ cup freshly squeezed
 orange juice
¼ tsp. salt (or to taste)
1 tsp. grated lemon rind

2 cups scraped and
 thinly sliced fresh
 young carrots
1 tbs. finely chopped
 fresh mint

Combine stock, orange juice, salt and lemon rind in heavy 10-inch skillet. Bring to a boil. Add carrots and stir them about a bit in the liquid. Then cover, reduce heat so that liquid barely simmers. Cook, shaking the pan occasionally, and checking to see whether the liquid has evaporated, in which case add a tbs. or so of stock or water.

The carrots should be tender in about 20 to 30 minutes and the liquid almost all evaporated. If not, boil it down a bit before pouring it over the carrots in a serving dish. Sprinkle with mint just before serving.

4 servings (about 30 calories per serving).

BRAISED TURNIPS

Another low-calorie vegetable that can add immeasurable flavor to a meat. Sturdy and filling, turnips can substitute for potatoes, thus reducing calories without reducing the meal's appetite satisfaction.

1½ lbs. small white
 turnips
½ cup fat-free chicken
 stock

1 tbs. Madeira
1 tsp. sugar
¼ tsp. salt

Peel turnips and cut them into quarters. Place in a single layer in a heavy 10-inch skillet (one with a tight-fitting cover). Add remaining ingredients and bring to a full boil. Cover skillet, lower heat so that liquid barely simmers and cook for 20 to 25 minutes, or until turnips are tender but not falling apart. Remove them to a serving dish. Boil down liquid remaining in skillet until reduced almost to a glaze. Pour over turnips and serve. 4 servings (about 75 calories per serving).

BRAISED ENDIVE

This is a rich-tasting vegetable that is especially good with roast turkey or chicken. Because endive is so calorie low—so low in fact that what calories they do contain are canceled out by the energy used in eating and digesting them—they can be enhanced by the flavor of butter and eaten without one bit of guilt.

8 Belgian endives	1 tbs. lemon juice
2 tbs. apple cider vinegar	2 tsp. sugar
½ tsp. salt	1 tbs. butter, very cold and cut into thin
½ cup fat-free chicken stock	slivers
	1 tbs. minced parsley

Trim the endive, slicing away as much of the root as possible without loosening the leaves.

Fill a large pot with water. Add vinegar and salt. Bring to a boil, add the endive, lower heat and simmer for about 10 minutes. Remove from the water with kitchen tongs and place heads side by side in a shallow baking dish just large enough to hold them.

Combine stock, lemon juice and sugar in a small saucepan; bring to a boil and pour over endive. Dot with butter slivers. Cover the baking dish with foil and seal. Bake in preheated 375° oven for 45 minutes to 1 hour.

To serve: Remove endive to a serving dish. Reduce cooking liquid in a small saucepan on top of stove to about 2 tbs., stir in parsley, pour over the endive and serve at once.

4 servings (about 30 calories per serving).

CASSEROLE OF BRAISED CABBAGE, POTATOES AND APPLES

1 medium head of green cabbage, cut in half and each half thinly sliced
3 California white (or other) baking potatoes, peeled and thinly sliced
3 large cooking apples (preferably greenlings), peeled, cored and thinly sliced

1 medium onion, finely chopped
Salt
Freshly ground black pepper
1 to 1½ cups fat-free chicken stock
¼ cup fine dry bread crumbs
¼ cup finely grated Swiss cheese

Preheat oven to 350°.

Arrange one-third of the cabbage, potatoes, apples and onion in a large well-buttered baking dish. Sprinkle with salt and pepper. Repeat with two more layers.

Pour in sufficient stock to come just below top layer. Cover dish and bake in preheated oven for about 45 minutes or until vegetables are tender. Sprinkle with bread crumbs and cheese. Return to oven and bake uncovered until the top becomes lightly browned.

Serves 6 to 8 (about 125 calories serving for 6; about 100 calories per serving for 8).

STIR-FRY, A GREAT WAY TO COOK VEGETABLES

Crisp texture, bright colors, conserved nutrients, terrific new taste and low-calorie count are what stir-fry vegetable dishes are all about. Simply slice or dice your vegetables and stir them fast in hot oil in a wok or a heavy skillet. Cover and steam a minute or so and serve. Try the following combinations or mix and match your own. All vegetables take to this low-calorie method of cooking.

For a super quick-to-the-table meal, serve slices of cold roast turkey, chicken or veal with a stir-fry medley of vegetables and freshly cooked, fluffy white rice. A little (bottled or homemade) chutney is a nice accompaniment and you can calorie afford it because, though the meal is high in appetite satisfaction, it is at the same time extremely calorie low.

STIR-FRIED CURRIED GREEN BEANS

1 lb. fresh green beans	½ tsp. salt
1 medium-size onion	¼ cup chicken stock
3 tbs. vegetable oil	1 tbs. lemon juice
1 to 2 tsps. Madras curry powder	Grated lemon rind (optional)

Wash beans, trim ends with a sharp knife. Slice diagonally into 1-inch-long bias slices.

Peel and chop onion.

Heat oil in a heavy skillet or wok. Stir in beans and onion. Cook, stirring constantly, for 2 to 3 minutes. Stir in curry powder and salt. Add stock and lemon juice. Cover and steam, stirring frequently, for about 8 minutes or until beans are crisp-tender. If desired, sprinkle each serving with grated lemon rind.

4 servings (about 135 calories per serving).

WINTER VEGETABLE STIR-FRY

1 small bunch white turnips	1 tsp. sugar
	½ tsp. salt
2 medium-sized carrots	¼ cup chicken or beef stock
2 or 3 stalks celery	
1 small green pepper	½ to ¾ cup bean sprouts (optional)
1 medium onion	
2 tbs. peanut oil	Soy sauce
2 to 3 drops sesame oil	

Peel turnips; cut into thin slices. Cut slices into "match sticks."

Scrape carrots: cut diagonally into thinest possible bias slices.

Trim celery; cut diagonally into bias slices about ½ inch long.

Wash pepper; cut in half, remove white fiber and seeds. Cut into "match sticks."

Peel and chop onion.

Heat oils in a wok or heavy skillet; add turnips, carrots, celery, green pepper and onion.

Stir-fry over medium-high heat for 3 to 4 minutes. Sprinkle with sugar and salt. Add stock. Lower heat, cover and steam, stirring frequently, for about 10 minutes or until vegetables are crisp-tender. (If liquid evaporates completely, add 2 to 3 tbs. stock but no more than necessary as vegetables should be almost dry when tender.)

Uncover. Add bean sprouts. Stir-fry for 30 seconds. Add soy sauce to taste and serve at once.

4 to 6 servings (75 and 100 calories per serving).

ITALIAN STIR-FRY EGGPLANT

1 green pepper
1 cucumber
¼ lb. mushrooms
1 small Bermuda onion
1 clove garlic
1 small eggplant (about ½ lb.)
1 large tomato
5 tbs. vegetable oil (or 2 tbs. vegetable oil and 3 tbs. olive oil)
½ tsp. salt
¼ tsp. pepper
1 tsp. mixed Italian herbs
2 tbs. minced parsley

Wash pepper, cut in half. Remove white fiber and seeds. Cut into very narrow strips.

Peel cucumber, cut in half lengthwise, and scoop out and discard seeds. Slice ¼ to ½ inch thick.

Wipe mushrooms clean with a damp cloth. Cut into quarters through stems.

Peel and chop onion. Peel and mince garlic. Combine.

Wash eggplant and dice into about ½-inch cubes. Do not peel.

Cut tomato in half horizontally. Squeeze out all seeds and juice (save the juice for soup if you like). Cut halves into thin, thin slices.

Heat 2 tbs. of the oil in a wok or large heavy skillet. Add the green pepper, cucumber, mushrooms, onion and garlic. Stir-fry over high heat for 4 to 5 minutes. Remove with a slotted spoon to a bowl.

Heat remaining oil in wok or skillet. Add eggplant. Stir-fry and toss for 4 to 5 minutes or just until tender.

Return cooked vegetables to pan. Add tomato. Sprinkle with salt and pepper and Italian herbs. Stir to blend. Cover and steam for 4 to 5 minutes. Stir in minced parsley.

Makes 4 to 6 servings (about 200 calories for each 4 servings; about 120 calories for each 6 servings).

STIR-FRY SPRING VEGETABLES

1 lb. asparagus	2 tbs. water
1 lb. fresh green beans	2 tbs. fresh lemon juice
1 fresh (not storage) carrot	Salt
1 small tomato	Pepper
3 tbs. vegetable oil	Minced parsley

Break woody ends from asparagus and discard. Wash stalks well under cold water, If sandy, cut off scales with the tip of a sharp knife, then wash stalks again. Cut off tips and set aside. Cut stalks diagonally into pieces about 1 inch long.

Wash beans. Trim ends with a sharp knife. Slice diagonally into 1 inch-long pieces.

Scrape carrot; cut diagonally into the thinnest possible ovals.

Cut tomato in half horizontally; squeeze out juice and seeds (reserve the juice to add to soups or stews if you like). Cut halves into thin strips about 1 inch long.

Heat oil in a large skillet or wok. Add sliced asparagus stalks, green beans and carrot. Stir-fry for 3 to 4 minutes. Add water. Cover and steam for 3 to 4 minutes. Uncover and continue to stir-fry until vegetables are just crispy tender. Add asparagus tips and tomato strips and stir-fry for 2 to 3 minutes longer. Add lemon juice, salt and pepper. Cover and steam for about 30 seconds. Uncover and stir-fry for a final 30 seconds.

Spoon into heated serving dish. Sprinkle with parsley and serve at once.

Makes about 6 servings (about 105 calories per serving).

STIR-FRIED PEAS, TINY WHITE ONIONS AND MUSHROOMS

1 small white onion
6 to 8 large fresh
   mushrooms
2 tbs. vegetable oil
2 lbs. fresh peas, shelled
   (2 cups)
8 tiny white boiled
   onions

½ cup homemade
   chicken stock
2 tsps. cornstarch,
   smoothed to a paste
   with 2 tbs. stock or
   water
½ tsp. salt (or to taste)

Peel and mince onion.

Wipe mushrooms clean with a damp cloth; trim stem ends. Cut through stems into thin slices.

Heat oil in a large skillet or wok. Add minced onion and mushrooms. Stir-fry for 3 minutes over medium-high heat. Add peas and stir-fry for 4 to 5 minutes or until peas turn a bright green. Add boiled onions and chicken stock. Cover and steam for 3 minutes longer.

Gently stir in cornstarch paste and cook, stirring, until liquid thickens. Season with salt.

Makes 4 servings (about 165 calories per serving).

STIR-FRIED BROCCOLI ORIENTAL

1 bunch fresh broccoli
   (about 1½ lbs.)
6 to 8 water chestnuts
3 tbs. peanut oil
2 to 3 drops sesame-
   seed oil
1 clove garlic, peeled
   and finely minced

4 tbs. white wine,
   chicken stock or water
2 tbs. soy sauce
½ tsp. sugar
Salt

Trim outer leaves and tough ends from broccoli; cut off flowerettes and set aside; slice stalks thinly.

Thinly slice water chestnuts.

Heat peanut oil and sesame oil in a heavy skillet or wok over medium-high heat. Stir in garlic and cook for 15 seconds. Add sliced broccoli stalks: Stir-fry for 4 to 5 minutes. Stir in water chestnuts, wine, soy sauce and sugar. Add flowerettes. Cover, lower heat, and, stirring once or twice, steam for 4 to 5 minutes, or until broccoli is crisp-tender. Season lightly with salt.

Serve with additional soy sauce to sprinkle over each serving.

4 to 6 servings (about 160 calories for each 4 servings; 100 calories for each 6 servings).

STIR-FRY SPINACH WITH BEAN SPROUTS

1½ lbs. fresh spinach	Freshly ground black
1 small onion	pepper
1 clove garlic	1 tbs. Madeira
2 tbs. vegetable oil	½ to ¾ cup bean sprouts
½ tsp. salt	

Remove stems from spinach.

Fill clean sink or a large pot with cold water. Dump in spinach leaves and swish them around. Sand and grit will loosen and drift to bottom. Lift out spinach and place in a colander to drain.

Peel and chop onion. Peel and mince garlic.

Heat oil in a large skillet or wok; add onion and garlic and stir-fry until soft. Add spinach, salt, pepper and Madeira. Cook, turning and stirring gently, for 2 to 3 minutes, or until spinach is wilted. Stir in bean sprouts. Serve at once.

4 servings (about 125 calories per serving).

PURÉE OF CELERY ROOT AND POTATOES

Mashed potatoes really made truly calorie low by being puréed with celery root and seasoned with chicken stock.

1 lb. celery root	2 lbs. new potatoes
Ice water	Salt
Juice of 1 lemon	Freshly ground black
Chicken stock (about	pepper
1½ cups)	

Peel celery root, cut into thin slices and chop slices. As you work, drop each chopped slice into a bowl of ice water mixed with the lemon juice. This will prevent discoloration. When all slices are chopped, drain, and place them in a large saucepan with sufficient chicken stock to barely cover. Cover the pan and place over low heat.

Peel and chop potatoes. Add them to the celery root after it has cooked for about 5 minutes. Cover and continue to cook—braise really—until tender. About 20 minutes. Uncover, increase heat and cook, stirring rapidly, until almost all liquid has evaporated. Drain, but reserve remaining liquid. Put through a ricer or food mill. Season to taste with salt and pepper, add a little of the reserved hot (reheat if necessary) cooking liquid and beat until smooth and fluffy.

Serves 6 (about 75 calories per serving).

PURÉE OF TURNIPS

2 lbs. small white	½ cup water
turnips	½ tsp. salt
1 tbs. butter	¼ tsp. pepper
1 tsp. sugar	

Wash and peel turnips. Coarse chop. Place in a medium saucepan with butter, sugar, water, salt and pepper. Cover and cook over low heat until very tender, about 30 minutes. Uncover, increase heat and cook, stirring often, until almost all liquid has evaporated. Remove from heat and, using a fork, mash to a smooth purée. If necessary, return pan to heat and cook, stirring until turnips are about the consistency of mashed potatoes.

Serves 6 (about 80 calories per serving).

PURÉE OF BUTTERNUT SQUASH

1 large butternut squash	Salt
⅓ cup beef stock	Pepper
1 tbs. Madeira	

Wash squash, peel and discard stringy inner portion and seeds. Coarse chop. Place in medium saucepan with stock and Madeira. Cover and cook over low heat until very tender, about 30 minutes. Uncover, increase heat and cook, stirring often, until almost all liquid has been absorbed. Remove from heat and mash with a fork. If necessary return to heat and cook, stirring, until thick-purée consistency has been reached. Season to taste with salt and pepper.

4 servings (about 50 calories per serving).

GREEN BEAN CASSEROLE

1 lb. fresh green beans
6 to 8 very small white onions
1 cup fat-free chicken stock
2 tbs. Crème Fraiche (see p. 102)
1 tbs. Parmesan cheese
1 tbs. fine cracker crumbs

Wash and trim the green beans. Place on a rack in a heavy skillet filled with about 2 inches of water and steam until just tender, about 10 minutes. Add more water if necessary. Peel the onions, cover with water in a small saucepan and simmer over medium heat until tender, about 30 minutes. Drain and combine with green beans in an ovenproof casserole. Combine stock and Crème Fraiche in the saucepan used for the onions. Slowly bring to simmering. Do not allow to boil. Cook, stirring, until sauce has thickened slightly. Pour over beans and onions. Sprinkle with cheese and crumbs and bake in a 350° oven until very hot and top is lightly browned, about 10 minutes.

Six servings (about 60 calories per serving).

POTATO-ONION CASSEROLE

This is a low-calorie version of an old favorite. Instead of milk and butter the recipe uses low-calorie, high-protein beef stock for added nutrition as well as extra flavor. Substantial enough to serve as a main course accompanied by a salad of crisp greens such as Bibb and Boston lettuce. Dessert could be honey-glazed apples with a spoonful of yogurt.

4 medium potatoes,
  preferably the thin-
  skin California
  potatoes
3 mild onions

1 tsp. butter
  Salt
  Freshly ground pepper
1½ cups beef stock

Preheat oven to 300°.

Scrub the potatoes well under cold running water. Do not peel, but slice as thinly as possible. Peel and cut the onions into thin slices; break into rings. Lightly grease a medium ovenproof casserole with the butter and fill with alternate layers of potatoes and onions, ending with a layer of potatoes. Sprinkle each layer very lightly with salt and pepper. Pour beef stock over potatoes and onions. Bake casserole in oven until potatoes are soft and most of the liquid has evaporated. About 1 hour.

Serves 6 (about 100 calories per serving).

BAKED POTATO CUBES

3 large Idaho potatoes
2 egg whites

1 tbs. water
  Salt

Preheat oven to 425°.

Peel potatoes, cut in half lengthwise and cut each half into 4 thick wedges.

Beat egg whites with water until blended. Roll each potato wedge in mixture and place on a rack (a cake rack does nicely) over a baking sheet. Sprinkle each lightly with salt. Bake in preheated oven for 30 to 40 minutes or until crisp on the outside, soft in center.

Serves 6 (about 55 calories per serving).

20
Salads and Dressings

SALADS—What miserable concoctions have been made under that name, but it need not be ever thus. A salad can be a fabulous meal in itself, a buffet party star or just about all things to all people—including the dieter—when it comes to good eating. No, you can't make a meal out of a few pallid slices of supermarket tomatoes on a bed of iceberg lettuce—but that's not a salad; that's a mess. Look to the Mediterranean countries for salad ideas that do make a meal.

For example:

MOROCCAN SALAD

2 cups cubed leftover cold roast lamb	1 tbs. chopped sweet pickle
2 cups cubed cold boiled new potatoes (leave skin on)	¼ cup mayonnaise
	2 tbs. lemon juice
	1 tsp. sugar
1 cucumber, peeled and chopped into cubes	2 heads Bibb lettuce
	12 ripe olives

Combine lamb, potatoes, cucumber and pickle in a large mixing bowl. Mix mayonnaise, lemon juice and sugar in a separate small bowl and beat with a wire whisk to blend. Pour over lamb and potatoes. Toss well. Refrigerate for 2 or 3 hours to allow flavors to mellow.

When ready to serve, line a salad bowl with Bibb lettuce leaves and pile meat-and-potato mixture in center. Garnish with ripe olives.

Serves six (about 300 calories per serving).

If this sounds like a high-calorie combination, it is not. Only the mayonnaise is really calorie-laden and ¼ cup for six servings adds up to very little per serving. This salad is, however, wonderfully "filling" and is rich in protein, vitamins and minerals. Delicious too.

TOMATO SPECIAL

1 head Boston lettuce	1 tsp. sugar
6 ripe tomatoes	1 cup cubed mozzarella cheese
Freshly ground black pepper	6 whole anchovies, each cut lengthwise into 2 thin strips
Salt	
¼ cup salad oil	
2 tbs. apple cider vinegar	

Wash, blot dry and separate lettuce leaves, discarding core, tear into bite-size pieces. Arrange on six salad plates. Peel tomatoes by dipping briefly into boiling water, then slip off the skins with the point of a sharp knife. Slice.

Start salad by placing one tomato slice on each plate, over lettuce. Sprinkle with freshly ground pepper and salt. Overlap with another tomato slice and repeat seasoning. Continue until all tomato slices are used.

Combine oil, vinegar and sugar in a small bowl. Beat well to blend. Spoon over salads and garnish each with mozzarella cheese cubes and anchovy strips.

Serves 6 (about 125 calories per serving).

SUMMER SALAD

1 head Boston lettuce
2 very ripe tomatoes, peeled, seeded and chopped
2 cucumbers, washed, trimmed and chopped (peel left on if cucumbers are unwaxed; the supermarket variety must be peeled)

2 ripe peaches, peeled and sliced
2 bananas, peeled and sliced
½ cup sunflower seeds
½ cup raisins
½ cup Poppy Seed Dressing (see page 209-10)

Wash lettuce, blot-dry, remove and discard core. Tear leaves into bite-size pieces. Place in large salad bowl. Add remaining vegetables and fruits. Sprinkle with sunflower seeds and raisins. Toss with Poppy Seed Dressing.

Serves 6 (about 100 calories per serving).

SALAD NIÇOISE

½ cup mild oil
   (safflower, corn or
   peanut)
1 tsp. Dijon mustard
1 tsp. sugar
¼ cup vinegar (top
   quality wine vinegar
   or apple cider vinegar)
1 2 to 2-½ oz. flat can
   anchovy fillets
6 to 8 medium-sized
   new potatoes
1 lb. fresh green beans

1 seven-oz. can oil-
   packed tuna fish,
   drained and broken
   up with a fork
   Lettuce leaves
½ small red onion,
   peeled, sliced and
   separated into rings
4 to 8 cherry tomatoes
2 hard-cooked eggs,
   quartered
4 to 8 pitted black olives

TO PREPARE DRESSING:

Combine in container of electric blender the oil, mustard, sugar, vinegar, four anchovy fillets and all the oil from the tin. Blend until smooth. Set aside.

Scrub potatoes clean under cold running water. Cook in simmering water to cover until tender but not falling apart. Peel and slice.

While potatoes are cooking, wash beans and snap off ends. Steam-cook in a covered 10-inch skillet until crisp-tender. About 10 minutes. Drain.

Pour dressing into a large bowl and re-blend with a fork. Add still warm sliced potatoes and green beans. Add tuna and toss with a fork until well mixed. Refrigerate until ready to serve.

Spoon mixture equally onto 4 lettuce-lined salad plates or 8 appetizer size plates. Top each serving with a few onion rings and garnish with cherry tomatoes, wedges of hard-cooked egg, black olives and remaining anchovy fillets.

4 servings as a main-course luncheon dish (about 380 calories per serving); 8 servings as a first-course appetizer (about 190 calories per serving).

BOUILLABAISSE SALAD

Expensive but elegant, a great salad for a summer luncheon party. Iced tea is the perfect beverage and thin wheat wafers the perfect "go-with."

1 cup chopped celery
1 lb. lump crabmeat (frozen or canned)
1 lobster tail, cooked, removed from shell and sliced into bite-sized pieces
1 lb. shrimp, boiled, shelled and deveined
1 tbs. lemon juice
¼ cup homemade mayonnaise

2 heads Boston lettuce
1 bunch watercress
1 tbs. minced chives
3 tbs. Vinaigrette Dressing (page 205)
2 tomatoes, peeled and quartered
2 hard-cooked eggs, quartered into wedges
8 large pitted black olives

Put celery in a bowl and pour boiling water over it. Let stand a few minutes. Drain and pat dry. Combine celery, crabmeat, lobster tail and shrimp. Add lemon juice and mayonnaise. Toss lightly to blend. Refrigerate, covered, for about 1 hour or until time to serve.

Wash lettuce, blot dry, tear into shreds. Wash watercress and blot dry, remove and discard tough stems. Combine and toss with Vinaigrette Dressing. Place on a long serving platter or in a salad bowl. Top with seafood mixture and garnish with tomato wedges, quartered hard-cooked eggs and olives.

8 servings (about 250 calories per serving).

RED SNAPPER SALAD

4 Belgian endives
1 three- to four-lb. poached red snapper or other firm-fleshed fish (see basic recipe for poached fish, page 136)
8 to 10 chopped pimiento-stuffed olives
1 tsp. Dijon mustard
¾ cup mild salad oil
¼ cup tarragon vinegar
Salt
Freshly ground black pepper
Boston lettuce

Trim endives and cut crosswise into ½-inch-thick slices.

Skin, bone and flake fish into good-size pieces.

Combine endive, flaked fish and olives in a bowl.

Stir mustard into oil in a small bowl. Add vinegar. Beat with a fork until blended. Season with salt and pepper.

Pour over endive and fish. Toss lightly to distribute dressing evenly.

Cover and refrigerate until chilled.

Drain and serve on crisp leaves of Boston lettuce.

Serves 4 (about 250 calories per serving).

CAESAR SALAD

If you use a light hand with the croutons, this makes a perfect and satisfying low-calorie luncheon. Serve with a glass of dry red wine and follow with a ripe peach for dessert. Dieting is not a spartan affair—or it shouldn't be. Good-tasting, satisfying meals can be low calorie as is this salad so you can afford the few calories in the croutons, cheese and oil.

1 head of Romaine or
  Boston lettuce
2 heads Bibb lettuce
4 tbs. salad oil
¼ tsp. dry mustard
¼ tsp. fresh black
  pepper
¼ tsp. salt

4 ozs. blue cheese
  Juice of 2 lemons
8 anchovy fillets
2 eggs, at room
  temperature
1 cup garlic croutons

Wash lettuce. Wrap in wet paper toweling and chill well.

Combine oil, mustard, pepper, salt, cheese and lemon juice. Blend well.

When ready to assemble salad, cut anchovies into bite-size pieces and add to greens.

Boil two eggs for just one minute—no longer.

Pour dressing over salad, then add the two eggs. Toss lightly but thoroughly. Top with croutons and serve at once.

4 servings (about 300 calories per serving).

DEVILED-EGG SALAD

A nicely filling but non-fattening luncheon, stuffed eggs are good eating if a little imagination is one of the ingredients.

8 hard-cooked eggs

Do you know the right way to hard-cook an egg? It's easy but there is a right way and a wrong way. First the eggs must be at room temperature or they will crack during the cooking process. Start the eggs in cold water and bring to simmering over medium heat. Simmer gently for 15 minutes. Remove from heat and cool under cold running water. Crack the shell and remove, still under running water. This procedure makes it easier to remove the shell and results in smooth perfect eggs.

Cut eggs in half. Remove yolks to a flat plate and mash to a smooth consistency with the following:

2 tbs. mayonnaise	2 tbs. finely minced
1 tbs. of chili sauce	sweet pickle
1 tsp. Dijon mustard	1 tsp. celery seed
3 or 4 dashes Tabasco	

Blend well and stuff egg-white "shells" with the mixture. Garnish with an anchovy strip or pimiento-stuffed green olive slices if desired. Serve on Boston lettuce leaves with whole ripe plum tomatoes.

2 stuffed-egg halves per serving (about 115 calories).

COOKED VEGETABLE SALAD SUGGESTIONS

Any number of vegetables are at their best when steamed until just tender, then marinated in Vinaigrette Dressing (page 205) and well chilled before serving. Some of the best are:

Asparagus	Cauliflower
Artichokes	Green beans
Broccoli	

All vegetables improve in flavor if they are steamed instead of boiled. Use a cake rack in the bottom of a heavy pot that has a cover. Pour in about 2 inches of water, place the vegetables on the rack. Bring to a boil, then lower heat to medium and steam until tender.

Artichokes take much longer than the other vegetables suggested above, about 30 to 40 minutes, so the water will have to be replenished every 10 minutes or so. The artichokes are done when a leaf will pull out easily.

Cauliflower requires the next longest time, so again the water level should be checked frequently.

Don't overcook any vegetables; they become limp and tasteless. As soon as they are cooked pour cold water over them to stop the cooking process. Place in a non-metal bowl and pour the marinade over them while still warm. Chill well. Drain before serving.

Any of these vegetables make an admirable cold first course for dinner or you can make a super luncheon platter with an assortment. Serve with Italian bread-sticks and indulge yourself with a meringue and fresh strawberries for dessert.

VINAIGRETTE DRESSING

1 cup salad oil
Juice of 2 lemons (or
¼ cup apple cider
vinegar)

¼ tsp. salt
¼ tsp. fresh black
pepper
1 tsp. sugar

Combine all the ingredients. Beat well with a wire whisk and pour into a Mason jar with a close-fitting lid. Chill well. Shake before using.

Makes about 1 cup (about 125 calories per tbs.).

TOMATO ASPIC SALAD

ASPIC:

1 cup water
1 onion, peeled and
  thickly sliced
1 clove garlic, peeled
  and cut in half
  lengthwise
2 envelopes unflavored
  gelatin

1¾ cups tomato juice
¼ cup lemon juice
½ cup unsweetened
  pineapple juice
2 or 3 dashes Tabasco
2 or 3 dashes
  Worcestershire

FILLING:

½ cup finely chopped
  celery
¼ cup minced green
  onion
¼ cup minced green
  pepper
½ cup peeled, cored and
  finely chopped tart
  apple

1 pt. skimmed-milk
  cottage cheese

Lettuce leaves
Mayonnaise
Yogurt

Combine water with onion and garlic in a small
saucepan and simmer over low heat for 10 to 15 minutes.
Strain, reserving ½ cup of the water. Discard onion and
garlic and pour the reserved water into a second saucepan. Cool. Sprinkle gelatin over surface. Stir over low
heat until gelatin has dissolved.

Add tomato, lemon and pineapple juices, Tabasco and
Worcestershire. Blend and pour into a chilled 3-cup ring
mold. Chill until firm.

Combine the filling ingredients and chill. Turn aspic

ring out onto a lettuce-lined platter, fill with cottage-cheese mixture and garnish with mayonnaise mixed half and half with yogurt.

4 servings (about 200 calories per serving).

AVOCADO MOUSSE
WITH GRAPEFRUIT SECTIONS

4 large ripe avocados or sufficient to make about 1½ cups mashed avocado	2 or 3 dashes Tabasco
	½ cup yogurt
	1½ envelopes unflavored gelatin
⅓ cup fresh lemon juice	1 cup water
1 tbs. onion juice	1 cup grapefruit sections
½ tsp. salt	

Peel and mash avocado with lemon and onion juice, the latter obtained by using a small grater to grate a peeled onion. Strain and discard onion pulp. Stir in salt, Tabasco and yogurt.

Sprinkle gelatin over water in a small saucepan and stir over low heat until dissolved. Add to avocado mixture and blend thoroughly.

Oil a 3-cup mold and rinse with cold water. Pour in avocado mixture and chill until firm. Unmold onto serving plate and surround with grapefruit sections.

Serves 6 (about 300 calories per serving).

FRENCH POTATO SALAD

4 large California white
   potatoes
2 cups white wine
   vinegar
½ cup Vinaigrette
   Dressing (page 205)
Boston lettuce leaves
Freshly ground black
   pepper
Cayenne pepper

Peel potatoes and slice lengthwise as thin as possible. (If you have a vegetable cutter, use it; if not, your sharpest, surest chef's knife will do.) Cut potato slices into finest possible shreds, about 1 inch long. Wash and drain.

In a large pot bring vinegar and 2 cups of water to a full boil. Add potato shreds a few at a time to keep liquid boiling. Boil 7 to 8 minutes or until they are crisp-tender (and no raw taste remains). Drain in a colander. Transfer to salad bowl, add Vinaigrette Dressing and toss to blend. Let stand at room temperature for 20 to 30 minutes so that flavor mellows.

Serve on lettuce leaves as a salad. Just before serving add a grinding from the pepper mill and sprinkle lightly with cayenne.

4 servings (about 400 calories per serving).

Potatoes can also be served as an accompaniment to cold meat.

SOME SUGGESTIONS FOR FRUIT SALADS

Almost any combination of fresh fruit makes a good fruit salad and nothing can be more refreshing or better for you. However, there are some selections that "go together" particularly well. Here are a few that you might enjoy plus a super dressing for fruit that transforms fruit salad into something "extra special":

Avocado Slices and Grapefruit Sections
Melon Ball Assortment (Watermelon, Honeydew, Canta-
  loupe)
Banana Slices, Fresh Peaches, Seedless Grapes
Fresh Pears Stuffed with Blue Cheese
Finely Chopped Apple and Celery (mixed with a bit of
  mayonnaise)
Cooked and pitted prunes (stuffed with cream cheese and
  sunflower seeds)
Orange Sections, Fresh Pineapple and Chopped Dates

Naturally you will dream up your own combinations
of whatever is fresh and in season. Cottage cheese is, of
course, the usual accompaniment to any fruit salad, but
if you find cottage cheese a bore, try mixing it with a few
dashes of Tabasco and a handful of toasted sunflower
seeds—added nutrition from the seeds plus lots more
flavor.

Because few people want dessert after a fruit-salad
lunch you can afford the calories of a watercress and
deviled-ham sandwich made with very thin sliced firm
white bread such as Pepperidge Farm or Arnold and
using just a trace of butter. Or have a wedge of creamy
Camembert or Brie cheese with a piece of crusty French
bread in place of a sweet dessert.

But dressing makes a fruit salad special and this is the
best one I know:

POPPY-SEED DRESSING

1 cup mild salad oil (not olive)   ½ cup honey
¼ cup fresh lemon juice   2 tbs. poppy seeds   Dash of salt

Combine oil, lemon juice and honey in a good-size
mixing bowl and beat with an electric mixer until thick

and well blended. If you don't have an electric mixer, a hand rotary beater will do the job; it just takes a stronger arm.

Add poppy seeds and salt and beat again. Cover and store in refrigerator until needed. If dressing separates beat briefly before using.

Makes about 1¾ cups (about 90 calories per tbs.).

PERFECT MAYONNAISE

Usually forbidden on most diets, mayonnaise, like a lot of other foods, is a much-maligned dieter's "no, no." Actually a small amount of mayonnaise made with unsaturated vegetable oil is beneficial in a weight-loss regime. Your body needs some oil to help burn up calories; it's animal fat that is the culprit. No, certainly you can't eat a cup of mayonnaise a day, but who wants to? A tablespoon on salad or mixed with finely shredded low-calorie cabbage in a delicious coleslaw that includes raw apples is not a dieter's sin but a benefit. Commercial mayonnaise is loaded with questionable additives, so the smart person who is health- and beauty-minded will make her own. It's easy, actually fun to do and it tastes superb.

2 egg yolks	3 tbs. wine vinegar or
½ tsp. dry mustard	lemon juice
¼ tsp. salt	1 cup vegetable oil such
1 tsp. sugar	as safflower oil
Pinch of cayenne	
pepper	

Beat the egg yolks in a small bowl until thick and lemon-colored. Add seasonings and 1 tbs. of the vinegar or lemon juice. Beat very well. Start adding the oil a teaspoonful at a time, beating thoroughly after each addition. This is easier if done with an electric beater, but it can be done with a wire whisk. As mixture thickens, the oil may be added a bit faster.

Finally add the remaining vinegar or lemon juice and beat again until well blended. Chill until ready to use. Mix with half yogurt, if you like, for a super-tasting dressing that is wonderfully good for you.

Makes about 1½ cups mayonnaise (about 90 calories per tbs.).

COTTAGE CHEESE

To make cottage cheese a lifelong friend to your figure, season one 8-oz. carton cottage cheese with salt, pepper and any of the following combinations:

(8 ozs. cottage cheese 240 calories plus additions)

3 tbs. crumbled Roquefort cheese
Dash Tabasco
about 50 additional calories

2 tbs. honey
1 tbs. fresh lemon juice
1 tbs. poppy seeds
about 70 additional calories

2 tbs. toasted slivered almonds
1 small tart apple, peeled, cored and chopped
about 150 additional calories

3 or 4 chopped stewed apricots or prunes
1 tbs. honey
1 tbs. lemon juice
about 75 additional calories

¼ cup yogurt prepared with any preserved fruit *about 65 additional calories*

2 tbs. chopped walnuts
2 tbs. chilled chopped cranberry jelly   *about 150 additional calories*

2 tbs. chopped mango chutney
1 tbs. juice from chutney
1 tbs. lemon juice   *about 100 additional calories*
Dash curry powder

4 slices shredded dry chipped beef
2 tbs. chopped celery   *about 50 additional calories*
1 tbs. minced green onion

¼ cup Vinaigrette Dressing (see page 205)
2 tbs. sunflower seeds   *about 50 additional calories*

2 tbs. toasted slivered almonds
1 tbs. honey   *about 100 additional calories*

½ cup peeled and grated cucumber
1 tbs. minced chives   *about 10 additional calories*

A "SPECIAL" ON YOGURT

I've mentioned yogurt so often throughout this book that it would not be complete without recipes for the homemade variety—for eating and for cooking as well as a "how to" for the mildest most delicious cheese you will ever taste, off or on a weight-loss diet. Neither elaborate equipment nor special skills are necessary in yogurt-making. It's easy, simple, inexpensive and the end product is so good for you you'll wonder how you ever lived without it always on hand.

HOMEMADE YOGURT

4 cups whole milk	2 tablespoons unflavored homemade or commercial yogurt (without preservatives)

Heat milk in a heavy medium saucepan until bubbles start to form around the side of the pan. Remove from heat. Beat yogurt until liquid, then stir it into the hot milk. Cover.

Heat oven to warm, then turn off heat. Let yogurt mixture stand in warm oven for 4 hours. Then reheat oven to warm, with door open. Turn off heat, close oven door, and let yogurt stand until it is thick.

Pour into four ½-pint jars. Refrigerate covered until needed. Will keep in refrigerator up to 2 weeks.

Makes 4 cups (about 150 calories per 1 cup).

YOGURT FOR COOKING

2 cups plus 2 tbs. unflavored homemade or commercial yogurt (without preservatives)	2 tablespoons cornstarch

Combine the 2 tablespoons yogurt with the cornstarch and blend well. Stir into remaining yogurt in a heavy medium saucepan. Bring to a simmer over low heat and cook, stirring often, for about 10 minutes or until thickened. Cool, pour into an electric blender and blend until smooth.

Makes about 2 cups (about 150 calories per cup).

YOGURT CHEESE

Place yogurt in a large sieve lined with a double thickness of dampened cheesecloth and set over a bowl. Let stand at room temperature for about 8 hours or until all liquid has drained off and the yogurt is firm. Season with salt to taste.

Makes about 2 cups (about 150 calories per cup).

21
Just Desserts

For most of us dinner simply doesn't seem complete without dessert. Luncheon seems all right without a sweet ending, but dinner? That's another story.

There is no reason, however, why the diet-bound diner can't have something delicious to end the meal. There are any number of dessert specials that use low-calorie ingredients—sponge and angel-food cakes, fruit of all kinds, creamy dessert cheeses that add protein along with great taste. There's no diet sin to any of them.

As with all food, keep the portions of dessert small and enjoy it with a small cup of fragrant black coffee to which has been added a spoonful of Cognac or Grand Marnier.

You will find Cognac and liqueurs such as Grand Marnier and kirsch a great help in transforming diet desserts into treats not treatments. A bowl of cold strawberries—sliced in half, sprinkled with just a trace of confectioners' sugar and a splash of Grand Marnier, then allowed to come to room temperature—is a taste experience that anyone, dieter or not, will find irresistible.

Super low-calorie grapefruit becomes appealing when broiled with a bit of brown sugar and given a tablespoon or so of kirsch while still warm.

In short, there's no need to deny yourself dessert on a

diet. It's *what* dessert that counts, not whether you have it or not.

YOU CAN HAVE YOUR CAKE AND DIET TOO

One of the reasons a lot of people can't stay on conventional diets is that they find it almost impossible to give up dessert and a broiled grapefruit simply doesn't always satisfy the habit of adding a sweet ending to a meal. Oh, sure I know you should give up sugar and I've said so earlier in this book, but if you hold your sugar intake to a very small amount, you can appease your sweet tooth without too much damage. One of the pleasantest ways to accomplish this happy balance is with sponge or angel-food cake. High in sweet-tooth satisfaction they weigh in very low on the calorie scale and, if served with puréed fresh fruit, they both become super desserts that you can easily afford on your calorie budget.

Next on the dieter's dessert list should be, of course, fresh fruit, but, if "just fruit" leaves you cold, try stepping up the taste quotient with a little imagination. Fresh strawberries or (if you are so lucky as to find them) raspberries, as well as fresh pineapple, are divine with a tablespoon of Grand Marnier Sauce (see recipe page 220). Or simply add a light sprinkling of sugar and a splash of Cognac or brandy, then allow the fruit to come to room temperature before serving.

Cooked fruit can end a meal perfectly too. For some reason cooked fruit seems like "more" than fruit served "as is," though the calorie count is not greatly increased. Try the recipe for Oranges in Spiced Wine (page 225), or Honey-glazed Baked Apples (page 219-20). Both are low in calories and high in "happy endings."

ANGEL-FOOD CAKE

The secret to a perfect angel-food cake is to beat the egg whites (they must be at room temperature) until really stiff, but not dry. They should stand in peaks when the beater is lifted out and should have a shiny, rather glazed, appearance. The best implement for this job is a French wire whisk. You simply cannot get the same volume with a rotary beater and air volume beaten into the whites is what makes or breaks an angel-food cake. Needed too, a light hand in folding the flour into the egg-white mixture. An over-and-under motion does the trick. Actually angel-food-cake is one of the easiest of all cakes to make and for the dieter it is indeed "heavenly."

12 egg whites, at room temperature	1½ cups superfine sugar
1½ tsps. cream of tartar	1 tsp. almond extract
	1¼ cups sifted cake flour

Preheat oven to 375°.

Beat egg whites until frothy. Beat in cream of tartar and continue beating until the egg whites form soft peaks. Gradually beat in 1 cup of the sugar and continue to beat until mixture is stiff enough to hold firm peaks. Fold in almond extract. Sift remaining sugar with flour and fold into egg whites gently but thoroughly. Pour into an ungreased 10-inch tube pan and bake for 35 minutes undisturbed. Check for doneness. Cake should be firm to touch and lightly browned.

Invert pan until cake is completely cold. Remove from pan and wrap in foil or plastic until ready to serve (about 150 calories per 3-inch slice).

Makes about 8 slices.

LEMON CHIFFON CAKE

If there comes a time in your dieting life where you simply cannot go on without a substantial dessert such as a piece of cake, and no piece of fruit will do, then make this big beautiful sponge cake. With less calories than any other (except angel food) cake and far less than pie, it is a superb ending to any meal. To make it even more delicious top each serving with a generous amount of puréed fresh strawberries or peaches.

2	cups sifted cake flour	5	egg yolks
1½	cups sugar	1	tbs. grated lemon rind
3	tsps. baking powder		Juice of one lemon
½	cup safflower, peanut or corn oil	½	cup water
		5	egg whites

Preheat oven to 325°.

Sift together the first three ingredients in a large mixing bowl. Make a well in the center and add the oil, egg yolks, lemon rind, lemon juice and water. Beat until mixture is very smooth and sugar has dissolved. Beat egg whites until stiff; fold gently into the batter. Pour into an ungreased 10-inch tube pan. Bake for 50 minutes, then increase heat to 350° and continue to bake for 10 more minutes. Invert and allow cake to cool before removing from pan.

About 10 servings (about 330 calories per serving).

MERINGUES

Are you dying for something really sweet for dessert? Yes, I know you want to cut out sugar, but a little doesn't hurt sometimes. So, if your sweet tooth is bothering you, make up a batch of meringues and have one—just one, with a serving of fresh fruit; peaches or strawberries are particularly good. If neither one is in season, unsweetened canned pineapple cut into chunks, is a good choice, or purée sliced pineapple in your blender. Meringues are much lower in calories than most desserts and are easy to make. They will keep well if stored in an airtight canister in a dry place. No, not refrigerated; they must stay dry or they become sticky and "weep."

6 egg whites	1 tsp. lemon juice
¼ tsp. salt	½ tsp. vanilla
1 cup sugar	

Preheat oven to 275°.

Allow the egg whites to come to room temperature before beating; they will beat up to a much higher volume than if beaten cold. Beat until they are quite stiff and the whites stand in peaks. Use a French wire whisk, not a rotary beater, for this job. While beating, gradually add salt and ½ of the sugar. Add lemon juice and vanilla and beat until mixture is very stiff. Add remaining sugar a tablespoon at a time, beating well after each addition.

Line a baking sheet with brown paper and drop meringues onto it with a tablespoon to form small balls. Bake in preheated oven for 45 minutes. When cool remove to airtight container.

Makes about 24 meringues (about 35 calories each).

HONEY-GLAZED APPLES

6 small tart apples	2 tbs. butter, melted
(McIntosh are best)	½ cup Cognac or brandy
1 cup honey	

Cut a slice from the top of each apple and scoop out core with a small spoon. Do not pierce bottom of apple.

Combine honey, butter and Cognac in a large baking dish that has a tight-fitting lid. Blend well. Add apples and spoon mixture over them. Place in a cold oven, adjust heat to 300° and bake, covered, for 30 minutes. Every 10 minutes uncover and baste with liquid. When soft, but still firm enough not to disintegrate, remove from oven and allow to cool, basting frequently with sauce. Serve at room temperature with sauce.

Serves 6 (about 275 calories per serving).

GRAND MARNIER
SAUCE FOR FRESH FRUIT

This is silken dessert sauce that has a gossamer smoothness simply too good to be believed. A tablespoonful over a serving of fresh fruit is a heavenly experience. Yes, it's high in calories, but, if used sparingly, it can cut your appetite for fattening desserts.

4 egg yolks	½ cup Grand Marnier
½ cup sugar	(Cognac or brandy
½ cup whipping cream	may be substituted)

Combine egg yolks and sugar in top half of a double boiler over—not in—simmering water. Beat constantly until very thick and pale yellow in color. Remove from heat and allow to cool to lukewarm.

Beat cream until stiff and fold into egg mixture. Add liqueur or Cognac a little at a time, beating as it is added. Refrigerate until served. Will keep up to a week if kept cold.

Makes about 2½ cups (about 115 calories per ¼ cup serving).

ORANGE CHAMPAGNE RING

4 envelopes unflavored gelatin	2 cups unsweetened pineapple juice
2 cups fresh orange juice	2 cups California Champagne
½ cup boiling water	

Soften the gelatin in ¼ cup of the orange juice in a large bowl. Add boiling water and stir until gelatin has dissolved. Add remaining orange juice, pineapple juice and champagne. Blend well. Pour into a ring mold that has been rinsed with cold water. Refrigerate until firm.

Unmold onto a serving platter. Fill center with fresh strawberries or sliced peaches if desired. To make this extra special serve with a small amount of Grand Marnier sauce (see recipe page 220.)

Serves 6 (about 100 calories per serving).

LIME MOUSSE

This is delicate, rich-tasting dessert while being very calorie low and low in sugar. Only ½ cup sugar for 6 to 8 servings.

6 eggs separated	1 tbs. grated rind of lime
½ cup sugar	
¾ cup freshly squeezed lime juice	1 envelope unflavored gelatin
1 tbs. butter	

Combine egg yolks, sugar, ½ cup of lime juice, butter, grated rind in the top half of a double boiler. Cook over simmering water until very thick.

Soften gelatin in remaining lime juice and add to egg

mixture. Stir until dissolved. Remove from heat and allow to cool slightly.

Beat the egg whites until very stiff and fold into custard. Pile into parfait dishes and chill until firm. Serve cold.

6 to 8 servings (about 170 calories for each of 6 servings; about 130 calories per serving for each of 8 servings).

COTTAGE CHEESE–PEACH "ICE CREAM"

1 10-oz. package of frozen peaches (or strawberries)
1 one-pint container low-fat cottage cheese

1 8-oz. container plain yogurt

Thaw frozen fruit until it can be broken up with a fork. Combine cottage cheese and yogurt in electric blender. Blend at high speed until smooth. If mixture seems too heavy add a small amount of milk (1 to 2 tbs.).

Combine thawed fruit with cottage-cheese mixture and mix well. Pour into 6 individual small molds and freeze. Unmold a few moments before serving.

Serves 6 (about 150 calories per serving).

FRESH PEACH ICE

6 cups fresh ripe peeled and coarsley chopped peaches
Juice of one orange
Juice of one lemon
½ to ¾ cup sugar (depending on ripeness and natural sweetness)

½ cup water
2 to 4 tbs. kirsch or light rum

Purée peaches in an electric blender or mash with a fork to a smooth purée.

Stir in orange and lemon juice.

Combine sugar and water and cook, stirring, over low heat until sugar dissolves. Combine with peach purée. Flavor with kirsch or light rum. Freeze in electric or manual ice-cream freezer as directed.

Serves 8 (about 115 calories per serving).

NOTE 1: You can also freeze this fruit mixture in ice-cube trays. Freeze to mushy stage. Transfer to a chilled bowl and beat until smooth.

Return to ice-cube tray and repeat. Just don't freeze until firm, but spoon at mushy stage into sherbet glasses and serve at once.

NOTE 2: You can substitute strawberries for the peaches and of course you can substitute artificial sweetener to your taste for the sugar syrup.

FRUIT CHAMPAGNE SHERBET

¼ cup fresh lemon juice	(slightly sweet) are
¾ cup fresh orange juice	actually an excellent
2 cups unsweetened	choice for this dessert
pineapple juice	1 tsp. grated lemon rind
2 cups champagne. The	½ package frozen
domestic brands	raspberries
labled Semi Sec	

Mix together everything but the raspberries. Put into a freezer tray and freeze to "mushy" stage. Stir to break up frozen particles. Repeat process several times, then heap into small bowls or parfait glasses.

Purée raspberries in an electric blender, spoon over sherbet and serve at once.

6 to 8 servings (about 80 calories per serving for 6 servings; about 50 calories per serving for 8 servings).

MELON COMPOTE

1 cranshaw melon	¼ cup kirsch
1 cantaloupe	1 tbs. sugar
½ small watermelon	

Any assortment of fresh melon may be used. The above gives a variety of taste and color. Cut with a melon baller. Place in a serving bowl. Sprinkle with kirsch and sugar. Cover and refrigerate until time to serve.

6 to 8 servings (about 125 calories per serving for each of 6 servings; about 100 calories per serving for each of 8 servings).

SPICED ORANGES AND WHITE GRAPES IN RED WINE

½ cup sugar	2 thin slices of lemon
½ cup water	6 large navel oranges
1 cup dry red wine	1 lb. seedless white
4 cloves	grapes
2 cinnamon sticks	

Combine sugar and water, wine, cloves, cinnamon and lemon in a medium saucepan and stir over medium heat until sugar dissolves. Bring to a boil, lower heat and simmer for 2 to 3 minutes to make a light syrup. Cool to lukewarm.

Peel, seed and slice oranges. Place in a serving bowl and cover with the warm syrup. Refrigerate until chilled. Just before serving add grapes to bowl.

Serves 6 to 8 (about 185 calories per serving for each of 6 servings; about 140 calories per serving for each of 8 servings).

BANANAS FLAMBÉ

4 firm bananas	4 tsps. sugar
4 tsps. butter	½ cup Cognac or brandy

Peel and cut the bananas in half horizontally, slice halves lengthwise into two pieces. Melt the butter in a heavy skillet or chafing dish, add the bananas, sprinkle with sugar and cook over medium heat for 5 to 10 minutes or until soft but not mushy. Add Cognac or brandy and cook only until liquid is hot. Ignite and bring, flaming, to the table. Serve as soon as flames die out.

Serves 4 (about 200 calories per serving).

Subject Index

pineapple, 51, 53
  with lemon or lime juice, 70
  with Perrier water, 70
  watermelon, 51

Kidneys, 81
Kirsch, 88, 102

Lactose, 50
Lamb, 81
  chops, 82
  calorie-protein ratio of, 62
Lard, 64
Laxatives, 27, 75
Lazlo, Ernst, 68
Lecithin, 65
Lemon juice, 56, 73, 75
Lemons, 75
  beauty care and, 75
  as seasoning, 86
Lettuce, 27-28, 59
Lillet, 107
Lime juice, 56
Liqueurs, 87-88
Liquor, 31-34, 58, 105
Liver, 81, 84
  calves, 61, 84
    sauce for, 88
  panbroiled, 83, 88
Lobster, 47, 48

Madeira, 87
Maltose, 50
Mangoes, 58
Mayonnaise, 49, 62
  yogurt, 25, 63
Melon, 28
Milk, 53
  in blender drinks, 78-79, 84
  as calcium source, 62-63
  skimmed, 62, 83
Mineral water, 51, 53, 56, 68-72
Minerals, 28-30, 32-33, 47, 50, 59
  in pill form, 30
Mountain Valley water, 69, 71-72
Mustard, 49, 88
Mustard greens, 59
Myths about dieting, 83-85

National Heart and Lung Institute, 48

Oatmeal, cosmetic use of, 75-76
Oils, 39
  unsaturated, 25, 28, 47, 64
    saturated vs., 28, 64
Onions, cocktail, 101

Orange juice, 56, 79
Oranges, 56
  poached in wine, 87
Organ meats, 28, 81, 168-69
Oysters, 100

Papaya, 58
Parmesan cheese, 58
Parsley, 25, 26, 86
  as vitamin C source, 56-57
Peaches, 28, 60, 82
Peanut butter, 49, 52
Peanut oil, 64
Pears, 25, 26
  poached in wine, 87
Pepper, 86, 101
Peppers, 47
Perrier water, 51, 56, 69-70, 105
Phosphorus, 62
Pickled herring, 101
Pineapple juice, 51, 53, 70
  with lemon or lime juice, 56, 73
  with Perrier water, 70
Pineapples, 28, 60
Plums, 60
Pork, 81
Potassium, 25-26
Potato chips, 29
Potato crisps, 105, 106
Potato straws, 48
Potatoes, 24, 25-26, 28, 50, 64, 82
  baked in skins, 57-58
  French fried, 93
Poultry
  as protein source, 61-62
  See also Chicken; Turkey
Protein, 25, 28
  bone, 25
  sources of, 60-66
Pumpkin, 59

Raspberries, 102
Riboflavin, 62
Rice, 64, 82
  parslied, 25
  wild, 101
Ricotta, 63
Ronsard, Nicole, 68
Roughage, 28

Safflower oil, 64
Salad, 84
Salmon, smoked, 101
Salt, 53-54
  substitutes for, 54
Sardines, canned, 61
Sauces, 88

Recipe Index